Pediatric Psychiatric Nursing

A Complete Evidence-Based Guide to Child and Adolescent Mental Health Assessment and Interventions

I0099748

Theo Seki

Table of Contents

Preface 1

Chapter 1: Overview of Pediatric Mental Health 6

The Current Mental Health Crisis 6

The Role of Pediatric Psychiatric Nursing 7

Historical Evolution and Current Challenges 9

The Evidence-Based Practice Framework 10

Emergency Department Vignette 11

Clinical Pearls 13

NCLEX-Style Questions 14

Chapter 2: Developmental Foundations Across the Lifespan ...17

Early Childhood (Ages 2-5) 17

School-Age (Ages 6-11) 19

Adolescence (Ages 12-18) 21

Neurodevelopmental Considerations 24

Developmental Milestone Tables 25

Brain Development Insights 26

Family Engagement Strategies Across Development 27

The Developmental Lens in Practice 27

Practical Applications 28

Developmental Understanding 28

**Chapter 3: Theoretical Frameworks and Therapeutic
Relationships 30**

Theoretical Foundations That Guide Our Work 30

Building Age-Appropriate Therapeutic Relationships 33

Family-Centered Care Approaches 35

Cultural Humility and LGBTQ+ Affirming Care 36

Putting It All Together 38

Real-World Refinements..39

The Healing Power of Relationships.............................39

Chapter 4: The Pediatric Psychiatric Assessment 41

The Biopsychosocial-Spiritual Framework....................41

Age-Appropriate Clinical Interviews 43

Mental Status Exam Modifications................................45

Risk Assessment and Safety Planning 47

Assessment Tools and Documentation 48

Real-World Assessment Challenges 50

Essential Takeaways for Practice..................................51

Chapter 5: Evidence-Based Screening and Assessment Tools...53

Early Childhood Tools (Ages 2-5)................................53

School-Age Instruments (Ages 6-11)............................55

Adolescent Screening (Ages 12-18)..............................57

Specialized Assessments..59

Tool Selection Strategies..60

Digital Platforms and Innovation 61

Integration with Clinical Practice.................................62

Practical Implementation Guide....................................63

Chapter 6: Diagnostic Formulation and Treatment Planning...65

DSM-5-TR Pediatric Adaptations.................................65

Case Formulation Models 67

Collaborative Treatment Planning 70

SMART Goals Development...71

Level of Care Determination...73

Treatment Matching and Sequencing 74

Documentation and Communication...75

Real-World Challenges and Solutions 76

Practical Application...77

Essential Principles for Success 78

Chapter 7: Psychotherapeutic Interventions Across Development 80

Early Childhood Interventions 80

School-Age Interventions...82

Adolescent Interventions..84

Specialized Modalities 87

Session Structure Across Development 89

Activity Guides and Engagement 90

Fidelity and Adaptation Balance..91

Real-World Implementation Challenges...................................91

Essential Practice Principles 92

Chapter 8: Psychopharmacology in Pediatric Populations........95

Pediatric Pharmacology Principles 95

Antidepressants and the Black Box Warning............................97

ADHD Medications 99

Antipsychotics and Metabolic Monitoring 100

Mood Stabilizers 102

Special Considerations..103

Practical Medication Management..105

Chapter 9: Crisis Intervention and Safety Management 108

De-escalation by Developmental Stage 108

Universal De-escalation Principles 110

Suicide Prevention and Safety Planning 111

Managing Aggressive Behavior Without Restraints.................114

Collaborative Crisis Management..116

Crisis Prevention Through Trauma-Informed Care 117

Technology in Crisis Management 118

Real-World Crisis Challenges..119

Post-Crisis Recovery...119

Building Crisis Resilience..120

Essential Crisis Principles...121

Chapter 10: Trauma-Informed Care and Complex Trauma ..123

Adverse Childhood Experiences and Developmental Trauma ..123

SAMHSA's Six Principles of Trauma-Informed Care...............125

Evidence-Based Trauma Interventions 128

Trauma-Focused Cognitive Behavioral Therapy (TF-CBT) 128

Special Populations and Unique Considerations......................131

Trauma Screening and Assessment Tools................................133

Environmental Factors and Healing Spaces.............................134

Self-Care Strategies for Providers...135

Implementation Challenges and Solutions...............................137

Working with Families in Trauma-Informed Ways..................138

Special Considerations for Different Age Groups 139

The Future of Trauma-Informed Care......................................141

Bringing It All Together...143

Chapter 11: Cultural Competency and Special Populations ...145

Cultural Competency Frameworks 145

Mental Health Disparities 147

Population-Specific Approaches...148

Racial and Ethnic Minorities..148

LGBTQ+ Youth..152

Foster Care Youth...154

Justice-Involved Youth..156

Homeless and Runaway Youth...157

Cultural Assessment and Intervention Strategies....................159

Building Cultural Bridges in Healthcare Settings....................161

Community Partnerships and Resources.................................163

Technology and Cultural Responsiveness 165

The Future of Culturally Responsive Care..............................167

Chapter 12: Family Systems and Parent Engagement............170

Family Systems Theory 171

Family Assessment Strategies...172

Evidence-Based Family Interventions 174

Parent Training and Support Strategies..................................178

Working with Complex Family Situations 180

Engaging Reluctant or Resistant Families 184

Supporting Diverse Family Structures....................................185

Family Communication and Problem-Solving Skills 187

Crisis Management in Family Systems....................................189

Technology and Modern Family Life 190

Working with Schools and Other Systems...............................192

Measuring Family Progress and Outcomes.............................193

Fostering Hope and Healing in Families.................................193

My Thoughts on Family-Centered Care 195

Chapter 13: Practice Settings Across the Continuum 196

The Continuum of Care Model 196

Inpatient Psychiatric Units 197

Outpatient and Community-Based Services 200

Intensive Outpatient and Partial Hospitalization Programs 202

School-Based Mental Health Services 204

Integrated Care Models 206

Telehealth and Digital Mental Health Services 207

Quality Indicators Across Settings 210

Team Roles and Interdisciplinary Collaboration 212

Transitions and Continuity of Care 214

Rural and Underserved Communities 216

Emergency and Crisis Services 217

Cultural Considerations Across Settings 219

Building a Better System of Care 220

Chapter 14: Legal, Ethical, and Regulatory Considerations ...223

The Legal Foundations 223

Consent and Assent in Pediatric Mental Health 225

Confidentiality with Minors 227

Mandatory Reporting Requirements 229

Additional Reporting Requirements 233

Involuntary Treatment and Hospitalization 234

Informed Consent for Treatment 235

Documentation and Record-Keeping 237

Ethical Decision-Making Frameworks 239

Professional Liability and Risk Management 240

Working with Special Populations 242

Quality Assurance and Regulatory Compliance 243

Technology and Legal Considerations 244

Building Ethical Practice...244

Chapter 15: Technology and Innovation in Pediatric Mental Health **247**

The Digital Generation and Mental Health.................................247

Telehealth in Pediatric Mental Health.......................................249

Digital Mental Health Tools and Applications 252

Social Media Impact on Youth Mental Health 255

Artificial Intelligence and Machine Learning 257

Virtual and Augmented Reality in Mental Health 260

Gaming and Gamification in Mental Health...............................262

Digital Divide and Equity Considerations 263

Privacy and Safety in Digital Mental Health 265

Emerging Technologies and Future Directions...........................266

Practical Implementation Guidelines 267

Balancing Innovation with Human Connection.........................268

Chapter 16: Professional Development and Leadership **271**

The Current State of the Pediatric Mental Health Workforce....271

Career Pathways in Pediatric Mental Health 273

Professional Certification and Credentialing 275

Continuing Education and Professional Development 277

Mentorship and Career Guidance...279

Leadership Development in Pediatric Mental Health 282

Research and Evidence-Based Practice 285

Self-Care and Resilience 287

Advocacy and Policy Engagement..290

Building Professional Networks 293

Entrepreneurship and Innovation 294

Preparing for the Future 296

Essential Tools for Success 299

References **302**

Preface

The journey that led to this book began over a decade ago when I first stepped onto a pediatric psychiatric unit as a newly licensed registered nurse. I thought I understood mental health care—after all, I'd completed my psychiatric nursing rotation and felt prepared to help children and families navigate their challenges. But nothing could have truly prepared me for the complexity, heartbreak, and profound hope I would encounter working with young people facing mental health crises.

My name is Philo G. Osei, and I am a registered mental health nurse with over a decade of practice in various mental health settings. From acute inpatient units to community mental health centers, from emergency departments to residential treatment facilities, I have witnessed firsthand both the devastating impact of untreated mental illness on children and the remarkable resilience of young people when they receive appropriate, evidence-based care.

During my years of practice, one thing became increasingly clear: there was a significant gap in educational resources specifically designed to prepare nurses for the unique challenges of pediatric mental health care. While excellent resources exist for adult psychiatric nursing and general pediatric care, the intersection of these specialties—caring for children and adolescents with mental health challenges—remained inadequately addressed in nursing education.

I've seen too many well-intentioned nurses struggle because they lacked the specialized knowledge needed to effectively assess a suicidal teenager, engage a traumatized child, or support a family in crisis. I've watched colleagues burn out not because they lacked compassion or clinical skills, but because they weren't adequately prepared for the emotional and clinical demands of this specialized practice.

This book emerged from those experiences and observations. It represents not just my own learning journey, but the collective wisdom I've gained from mentors, colleagues, and most importantly, from the children and families who have trusted me with their stories and their healing.

Throughout my career, I have worked across diverse settings that have shaped my understanding of pediatric mental health care. In acute inpatient units, I learned the critical importance of rapid assessment and crisis stabilization. In community mental health centers, I discovered the power of long-term therapeutic relationships and family engagement. In emergency departments, I witnessed the urgent need for skilled psychiatric nurses who could provide compassionate care during the most frightening moments of a child's life. My experience in criminal justice services opened my eyes to the complex intersection of mental health challenges and legal system involvement, where many young people cycle through detention facilities without receiving adequate mental health treatment. Working in forensic settings taught me the specialized skills needed to assess and treat adolescents who have both mental health needs and legal complications, often requiring careful coordination between therapeutic goals and court requirements. These forensic experiences highlighted how trauma, untreated mental illness, and systemic failures can lead young people into the justice system, reinforcing my belief that early intervention and comprehensive mental health services are not just clinical imperatives but also matters of social justice.

Each setting taught me something different about the complexity of mental health challenges in young people. A 7-year-old's anxiety manifests differently than a 17-year-old's depression. A family's cultural background profoundly influences how they understand and respond to mental health symptoms. The trauma that one child experiences as devastating, another child might process with remarkable resilience.

These experiences convinced me that pediatric mental health nursing requires specialized knowledge, skills, and approaches that go far beyond what is typically covered in general nursing education. We need nurses who understand child development and can adapt their communication style for a frightened 5-year-old versus an angry teenager. We need providers who can recognize the signs of trauma and respond in ways that promote healing rather than re-traumatization. We need professionals who can work effectively with families, understanding that parents and caregivers are often dealing with their own stress, guilt, and confusion about their child's mental health challenges.

This book is designed to fill that educational gap. It provides the comprehensive foundation that nursing students, new graduates, and practicing nurses need to deliver skilled, evidence-based care to children and adolescents with mental health challenges. But it's not just about clinical skills—it's also about understanding the broader context in which these challenges occur and the systems that either support or hinder recovery.

My goal in writing this text was to create the resource I wish I'd had when I began my career in mental health. I wanted to provide not just the theoretical knowledge that's essential for safe practice, but also the practical wisdom that comes from years of experience working with young people and their families.

Throughout these pages, you'll find case examples drawn from my practice experience (with all identifying information changed to protect privacy and confidentiality). You'll discover evidence-based interventions that have been proven effective in helping children and adolescents heal from mental health challenges. You'll learn about the legal and ethical considerations that are unique to working with minors. Most importantly, you'll gain an understanding of how to provide care that honors the dignity, strength, and potential of every child and family you serve.

The field of pediatric mental health is at a critical juncture. The need for services has never been greater, with rates of depression, anxiety, and suicidal ideation among young people reaching crisis levels. At the same time, we face significant shortages of qualified mental health professionals, particularly those trained to work specifically with children and adolescents.

But within this crisis lies tremendous opportunity. Nurses are uniquely positioned to help address this shortage. We are trained in holistic, family-centered care. We understand the importance of therapeutic relationships. We are skilled in assessment, intervention, and advocacy. With appropriate education and training, nurses can become powerful agents of healing for children and families facing mental health challenges.

This book is my contribution to preparing the next generation of pediatric mental health nurses. It represents years of clinical practice, extensive research into current evidence, and collaboration with colleagues across multiple disciplines and practice settings. But most importantly, it represents hope—hope that we can do better for the children and families we serve, hope that we can create more effective and compassionate systems of care, and hope that the nurses who read this book will be inspired to make pediatric mental health their calling.

The work is not easy. It requires emotional resilience, clinical expertise, cultural humility, and a commitment to ongoing learning and growth. But it is also profoundly rewarding. There is no greater privilege than being trusted with a child's pain and participating in their healing journey. There is no more important work than helping young people develop the skills and support they need not just to survive their challenges, but to thrive despite them.

As you read this book and consider your role in pediatric mental health care, I encourage you to approach this work with both confidence and humility. Be confident in the knowledge and skills you're developing, but remain humble about how much there is still to learn. Be passionate about making a difference, but realistic about the challenges you'll face. Most importantly, never lose sight of the fundamental truth that guides all good nursing practice: every child deserves to be seen, heard, valued, and supported in their journey toward healing and growth.

The children and families waiting for our care deserve our very best efforts. This book is designed to help you provide that level of care, but your commitment to ongoing learning, professional growth, and compassionate practice will ultimately determine the difference you make in their lives.

Theo Seki RMN
Registered Mental Health Nurse

Chapter 1: Overview of Pediatric Mental Health

You're stepping into pediatric psychiatric nursing at a time when young people need mental health support more than ever before. The statistics paint a sobering picture - nearly one in three adolescents will experience an anxiety disorder before they turn eighteen. Depression affects about 20% of teenagers. And these numbers keep climbing year after year.

This isn't just about statistics though. Behind every number is a child struggling to make sense of their emotions, a teenager feeling overwhelmed by life, or a family desperately seeking help for their little one. As a pediatric psychiatric nurse, you'll be on the front lines of this crisis, equipped with the knowledge and skills to make a real difference in these young lives.

The youth mental health landscape has shifted dramatically over the past decade, and understanding these changes is essential for providing effective care. We're not dealing with the same challenges our predecessors faced twenty years ago. Today's young people navigate a world of social media pressures, academic stress that starts earlier than ever, family structures that look different from previous generations, and yes, the lingering effects of a global pandemic that disrupted their most formative years.

The Current Mental Health Crisis

The scope of youth mental health challenges today is staggering. About 7.1% of children aged 3-17 have diagnosed anxiety, while 3.2% have diagnosed depression. But here's what makes these numbers even more concerning - many experts believe we're only seeing the tip of the iceberg. For every child receiving treatment, there are likely two or three more struggling in silence.

Suicide has become the second leading cause of death among people aged 10-14. Think about that for a moment. Children who should be worried about homework and friendships are instead battling thoughts of ending their lives. The suicide rate for this age group has increased by over 60% in the last decade. Among teenagers aged 15-19, the statistics are equally troubling, with suicide attempts among girls increasing by 51% between 2019 and 2021.

What's driving this crisis? There's no single answer, but several factors converge to create a perfect storm. Academic pressure starts younger than ever, with standardized testing beginning in elementary school. Social media creates constant comparison and fear of missing out. Many families struggle economically, adding stress to household environments. And perhaps most significantly, there's still tremendous stigma around mental health that prevents many young people from seeking help.

The COVID-19 pandemic acted as an accelerant to existing mental health challenges. During the height of lockdowns, emergency department visits for mental health crises among adolescents increased by over 30%. But even as restrictions lifted, the mental health impacts lingered. Young people missed crucial developmental experiences - first school dances, sports seasons, graduation ceremonies. They spent formative years isolated from peers, learning through screens instead of in-person connections.

Now we're seeing what researchers call "pandemic cohorts" - groups of children who spent critical developmental periods in isolation. A five-year-old who spent ages three to five in lockdown missed vital socialization opportunities. A teenager who started high school virtually struggled to develop normal peer relationships. These experiences have created unique mental health needs that we're still learning how to address.

The Role of Pediatric Psychiatric Nursing

As a pediatric psychiatric nurse, you occupy a unique position in the mental health care system. You're not just administering medications or monitoring vital signs - though those tasks matter too. You're building relationships with young people at their most vulnerable moments, serving as a bridge between medical treatment and emotional healing.

Your scope of practice encompasses assessment, diagnosis collaboration, treatment planning, medication management, therapeutic interventions, family education, and crisis intervention. But beyond these clinical responsibilities, you serve as an advocate, educator, and often, a beacon of hope for families navigating the complex mental health system.

In the inpatient setting, you might be the professional who spends the most time with a young patient. While doctors make brief rounds and therapists see patients for scheduled sessions, you're there during the 2 AM nightmare, the mealtime struggle, the visiting hour meltdown. You observe patterns others might miss. You notice when a typically chatty teenager becomes withdrawn, or when a child's anxiety peaks during certain activities.

Your role extends into various settings - emergency departments where you perform urgent assessments, outpatient clinics where you provide ongoing medication management, schools where you consult on behavioral interventions, and residential facilities where you help create therapeutic environments. Each setting demands different skills, but the core remains constant: you're there to help young people and their families navigate mental health challenges.

The therapeutic relationship you build with young patients differs fundamentally from adult psychiatric nursing. Children and adolescents rarely self-refer for mental health treatment. They're usually brought by concerned parents, referred by schools, or mandated by courts. This means you often start with a reluctant, possibly hostile patient who sees you as part of the adult system trying to control them.

Building trust with these young people requires patience, authenticity, and often, a willingness to meet them where they are.

This might mean discussing their favorite video game before addressing their depression, or allowing them to draw while talking about their anxiety. You learn to read between the lines - understanding that "I'm fine" might mean anything but fine, and that anger often masks fear or sadness.

Historical Evolution and Current Challenges

Pediatric psychiatric nursing is a relatively young specialty. For much of history, children with mental health issues were either hidden away by families, institutionalized in adult facilities, or simply labeled as "bad" children deserving punishment rather than treatment. The field really began taking shape in the 1940s and 1950s, influenced by pioneers who recognized that children's mental health needs differed fundamentally from adults'.

The introduction of child guidance clinics in the early 20th century marked a shift toward recognizing childhood mental health as distinct from adult psychiatry. These clinics brought together psychiatrists, psychologists, and social workers - but nurses were notably absent from early multidisciplinary teams. It wasn't until the 1960s that psychiatric nurses began specializing in pediatric populations.

The Community Mental Health Act of 1963 revolutionized mental health care delivery, moving treatment from large institutions to community settings. This shift created new roles for nurses, who became essential in delivering care in outpatient clinics, schools, and homes. The 1970s and 1980s saw the emergence of child and adolescent psychiatric nursing as a recognized specialty, with the first certification exam offered in 1979.

But even with this progress, we face significant workforce challenges today. The Health Resources and Services Administration projects we'll need 118,600 new psychiatric mental health nurse practitioners by 2036 just to meet current demand. Yet many nursing programs offer minimal pediatric psychiatric content.

9

Most BSN graduates receive perhaps one or two lectures on child mental health during their entire education.

The average age of psychiatric mental health nurse practitioners is 54, with about 25% planning to retire within the next six years. This looming retirement wave threatens to worsen an already critical shortage. Meanwhile, demand continues growing. More parents recognize mental health symptoms in their children. Schools increasingly refer students for evaluation. Pediatricians, overwhelmed by mental health concerns in primary care, desperately need psychiatric nursing support.

Geographic disparities compound these challenges. While urban areas might have several child psychiatrists and psychiatric nurses, rural communities often have none. Ninety-six percent of U.S. counties face mental health prescriber shortages. For many families, the nearest pediatric psychiatric nurse might be hours away, making regular treatment virtually impossible.

The workforce challenges extend beyond mere numbers. Pediatric psychiatric nursing demands specialized knowledge that many nurses lack. Understanding psychopharmacology in developing brains differs vastly from adult medication management. Recognizing age-appropriate behaviors versus pathological symptoms requires developmental expertise. Working with family systems adds layers of complexity not present in adult psychiatric care.

The Evidence-Based Practice Framework

Modern pediatric psychiatric nursing rests on a foundation of evidence-based practice. This means integrating the best available research evidence with clinical expertise and patient values. But in pediatric mental health, "evidence" often looks different than in other medical fields.

We can't always conduct randomized controlled trials with vulnerable child populations. Ethical considerations limit our ability

10

to withhold treatment from control groups. Long-term outcome studies are challenging when following children through developmental changes. So we rely on various forms of evidence - systematic reviews, cohort studies, expert consensus guidelines, and yes, clinical wisdom accumulated over decades of practice.

The evidence base for pediatric psychiatric interventions continues evolving. We know cognitive-behavioral therapy effectively treats adolescent depression. Trauma-focused CBT helps children process traumatic experiences. Family-based treatment shows promise for eating disorders. But we also recognize gaps in our knowledge. What works for a suburban white teenager might not translate to an urban Latino adolescent or a rural Native American child.

Evidence-based practice in pediatric psychiatric nursing means staying current with research while remaining flexible enough to adapt interventions to individual needs. It means recognizing that a seven-year-old's depression looks different from a seventeen-year-old's. It means understanding that cultural background influences how symptoms manifest and how families engage with treatment.

You'll use standardized assessment tools validated for specific age groups - the PHQ-9 modified for adolescents, the SCARED for anxiety disorders, the Vanderbilt for ADHD. But you'll also trust your clinical judgment when a child doesn't fit neatly into diagnostic categories. You'll follow medication guidelines while recognizing that pediatric psychopharmacology often involves off-label prescribing based on clinical experience rather than FDA approvals.

Emergency Department Vignette

Sarah, a 14-year-old, arrives at the emergency department at 11 PM on a Tuesday night. Her parents found her in her bedroom with superficial cuts on her forearm and empty pill bottles scattered on her bed - though it appears she hadn't ingested any. This is her third ED visit in two months.

As the pediatric psychiatric nurse, you enter Sarah's room to find her curled on the gurney, facing away from the door. Her mother sits in the corner, tears streaming down her face, while her father paces by the window, clearly frustrated.

"I don't want to talk," Sarah mutters before you even introduce yourself.

You pull up a chair - not too close, giving her space. "That's okay. You don't have to talk right now. I'm Jamie, one of the nurses here. I'll be checking in with you tonight."

Twenty minutes later, after sitting quietly and occasionally commenting on the late-night TV show playing, Sarah turns slightly toward you. "My parents think I'm crazy."

"That sounds really hard, feeling like your parents don't understand what you're going through."

She nods, tears starting to fall. "They keep saying I have everything - good grades, nice friends, all this stuff. They don't get that none of it matters when you feel empty inside."

This moment - this tiny opening - is where pediatric psychiatric nursing begins. Not with medications or formal assessments, but with connection. With showing a young person that someone will sit with them in their pain without judgment, without immediately trying to fix everything.

Over the next two hours, you learn about Sarah's perfectionism, her fear of disappointing everyone, her exhaustion from maintaining a perfect facade. You assess her safety, collaborate with the psychiatrist on admission decisions, comfort her parents, and begin building the therapeutic relationship that might, just might, be the turning point in this young person's life.

Clinical Pearls

Building Rapport with Reluctant Adolescents: Start with neutral topics before addressing mental health concerns. Comment on their shoes, ask about their music preferences, or notice something unique about them. Authenticity matters more than technique - young people have excellent radar for adults trying too hard.

The Parent Paradox: Parents are usually both your greatest asset and biggest challenge in pediatric psychiatric nursing. They provide crucial history and support, but their anxiety can overwhelm the therapeutic process. Learn to validate parent concerns while maintaining appropriate boundaries. Sometimes the most therapeutic intervention is helping parents manage their own emotional responses.

Developmental Context is Everything: A six-year-old expressing suicidal thoughts requires different assessment than a sixteen-year-old. Young children might not understand death's permanence but still experience genuine distress. Adolescents might minimize serious intent while secretly planning. Always assess within developmental context, not just chronological age.

The Medication Talk: Many parents fear psychiatric medications will "change" their child or create addiction. Address these concerns directly. Explain how medications work in developing brains, discuss both benefits and risks honestly, and emphasize that medication is often just one part of a comprehensive treatment plan. Use analogies they understand - like insulin for diabetes or glasses for vision problems.

Crisis Doesn't Always Look Like Crisis: The quietly withdrawn child might be in more danger than the one acting out dramatically. Learn to recognize subtle warning signs - giving away possessions, sudden mood improvement after deep depression, indirect goodbye statements. Your clinical intuition, developed through experience, becomes invaluable in recognizing these quiet emergencies.

NCLEX-Style Questions

1. A 15-year-old patient tells you they've been feeling "empty and numb" for the past three months. They maintain good grades but report having no energy or interest in previously enjoyed activities. Which assessment tool would be most appropriate for evaluating their symptoms?
   - A) CRAFFT screening tool
   - B) PHQ-9 modified for adolescents
   - C) Vanderbilt ADHD rating scale
   - D) CAGE questionnaire
2. You're admitting an 8-year-old to the inpatient psychiatric unit. The child appears frightened and keeps asking for their stuffed animal. What's your priority nursing intervention?
   - A) Explain the unit rules and schedule immediately
   - B) Complete the admission assessment as quickly as possible
   - C) Allow the child to keep their stuffed animal and orient them gradually
   - D) Contact the physician for sedation orders
3. During evening rounds, you notice a typically social 13-year-old patient sitting alone, hood up, refusing dinner. They were laughing with peers at lunch. What's your best initial response?
   - A) Document the behavior and continue rounds
   - B) Insist they join the group for dinner
   - C) Sit nearby and gently check in about their day
   - D) Call their parents to report the change
4. A parent demands you tell them everything their 16-year-old discusses in therapy sessions. How do you respond?
   - A) Explain confidentiality laws while acknowledging their concern
   - B) Share everything since parents have full access rights
   - C) Refuse to discuss anything about their child's treatment
   - D) Refer them to administration

5. You're teaching a newly diagnosed ADHD patient and family about stimulant medication. The parent asks, "Won't this just make them addicted to drugs?" Your best response includes:
   o A) "These medications are completely safe with no addiction risk"
   o B) "When taken as prescribed, ADHD medications actually reduce future substance abuse risk"
   o C) "All medications carry risks, but ADHD is worse"
   o D) "Your child is too young to become addicted"

The landscape of pediatric mental health continues evolving rapidly. New challenges emerge - social media impacts, vaping-related anxiety, climate change distress - while old stigmas slowly crumble. As a pediatric psychiatric nurse, you're entering this field at a pivotal moment. The need has never been greater, but neither has our understanding of effective interventions.

You'll witness heartbreak - young lives lost to suicide, families torn apart by mental illness, children bearing trauma no one should experience. But you'll also witness remarkable resilience. You'll see teenagers learn to manage their depression, anxious children find their courage, and families heal together. You'll be the steady presence during someone's darkest moment and celebrate with them when light returns.

This work isn't easy. It demands clinical expertise, emotional intelligence, cultural sensitivity, and endless patience. Some days you'll question whether you're making any difference at all. But then a former patient sends a graduation announcement, or a parent thanks you for saving their child's life, and you remember why this work matters so profoundly.

The young people you serve today will shape tomorrow's world. By helping them navigate their mental health challenges now, you're not just treating illness - you're nurturing future leaders, creators, parents, and healers. That's the true landscape of pediatric mental health nursing: one child, one family, one moment of connection at a time, building toward a healthier future for all.

Chapter 2: Developmental Foundations Across the Lifespan

Walking into a pediatric psychiatric unit for the first time, you might notice something striking - the dramatic differences between your patients. In one room, a five-year-old builds elaborate block towers while explaining how the "worry monster" visits at bedtime. Next door, an eleven-year-old meticulously organizes their belongings, anxious about returning to school after a panic attack. Down the hall, a seventeen-year-old scrolls through their phone, simultaneously texting friends and struggling with self-harm urges.

Each of these young people experiences mental health challenges, but their developmental stage shapes everything - how symptoms manifest, how they understand their experiences, what interventions work, and how you'll build therapeutic relationships with them. Understanding child development isn't just helpful in pediatric psychiatric nursing; it's absolutely essential.

Early Childhood (Ages 2-5)

These early years lay the groundwork for all future mental health. Young children between ages two and five exist in a world where fantasy and reality intertwine, where emotions feel enormous and overwhelming, and where their primary relationships shape their entire sense of safety and self.

Attachment forms the cornerstone of early childhood mental health. When a three-year-old consistently turns to their caregiver for comfort and receives responsive, warm attention, they develop secure attachment. This doesn't mean perfect parenting - it means "good enough" parenting where the child's needs are generally met with consistency and care. These securely attached children develop an internal working model that says, "I'm worthy of love, and others can be trusted to help me."

But what happens when attachment goes awry? You'll see it in the preschooler who can't be comforted, who either clings desperately or shows no preference for caregivers over strangers. These attachment disruptions often stem from early trauma, neglect, inconsistent caregiving, or parental mental illness. A four-year-old who experienced multiple foster placements might struggle to trust any adult, viewing relationships as temporary and unreliable.

Emotional regulation in early childhood looks nothing like adult emotional control. A preschooler's prefrontal cortex - the brain's control center - is still under major construction. When a four-year-old has a meltdown over a broken cookie, they're not being manipulative or dramatic. Their brain literally cannot yet regulate the tidal wave of disappointment flooding their system.

This is where co-regulation becomes crucial. Young children learn to manage emotions by borrowing their caregiver's calm nervous system. When you stay regulated while a preschooler tantrums, speaking in soothing tones and offering comfort, you're literally teaching their brain how to calm down. Over thousands of these interactions, children internalize this regulation ability.

Play serves as the primary language of early childhood. Through play, young children process experiences, express emotions, and practice social skills. Watch a four-year-old in the dollhouse corner of a psychiatric unit - they might reenact their parents' fights, their own hospitalization, or their fears about going home. This isn't just cute; it's therapeutic processing in action.

In your nursing practice, you'll use play therapeutically. Simple puppet shows help children express feelings they can't verbalize. Drawing activities reveal inner experiences - the family portrait where daddy is a tiny figure in the corner, or the self-portrait covered in black scribbles. Even medical play, letting children give "shots" to stuffed animals, helps them process their own medical trauma.

The magical thinking characteristic of this age creates unique challenges and opportunities. A three-year-old might believe their angry thoughts caused mommy's car accident. A five-year-old might think taking medicine will turn them into someone else entirely. These beliefs aren't delusions requiring antipsychotics - they're normal developmental phenomena requiring gentle clarification and reassurance.

Language development dramatically impacts mental health expression in early childhood. A two-year-old with limited vocabulary might bite when frustrated, not out of aggression but from inability to say, "I'm overwhelmed and need space." By age five, most children can verbally express basic emotions, though they still struggle with complex feelings like ambivalence or jealousy mixed with love.

You'll need to adjust your communication style dramatically for this age group. Forget long explanations about medication benefits. Instead, try: "This medicine helps your brain feel less worried, like putting on a cozy blanket when you're cold." Use concrete, sensory language they can grasp. Show rather than tell whenever possible.

The family system holds paramount importance in early childhood mental health. A preschooler's symptoms often reflect family dysfunction more than individual pathology. The anxious four-year-old might be responding to parental conflict. The aggressive five-year-old might be modeling witnessed violence. Always assess and treat within the family context at this age.

School-Age (Ages 6-11)

Something shifts around age six. Children enter what Piaget called "concrete operations" - they can think logically about concrete events, though abstract reasoning remains limited. This cognitive leap coincides with entering formal schooling, expanding peer relationships, and developing a sense of competence or inadequacy that can last a lifetime.

The school-age child's world expands beyond family to include teachers, peers, and community. Suddenly, they're comparing themselves to others constantly. "Why can Tommy read better than me?" "How come Sarah has more friends?" This social comparison drives either developing competence ("I'm good at math!") or feelings of inferiority ("I'm the dumbest kid in class").

Academic struggles and mental health intertwine significantly during these years. The eight-year-old with undiagnosed ADHD doesn't just struggle with attention - they internalize messages about being lazy, careless, or stupid. By fourth grade, they might develop secondary depression or anxiety. What started as a neurodevelopmental difference becomes a mental health crisis through repeated failure experiences.

Peer relationships take on enormous importance, yet social skills vary wildly. Some seven-year-olds navigate playground politics smoothly while others struggle with basic interaction. Social rejection during school-age years predicts later mental health problems more strongly than almost any other factor. The child eating alone every day at lunch isn't just lonely - they're at significant risk.

In your nursing role, you'll often see school-age children whose mental health symptoms first manifest as school problems. The nine-year-old refusing school might have separation anxiety, social anxiety, depression, or trauma responses to school-based bullying. Careful assessment reveals what drives the behavior.

Cognitive behavioral therapy works particularly well for school-age children because they can understand cause-and-effect relationships. A ten-year-old can grasp that thoughts influence feelings and behaviors. They can complete thought logs, practice coping skills, and engage in behavioral experiments. "So you think everyone will laugh if you raise your hand? Let's test that hypothesis."

But remember - concrete thinking still dominates. Abstract concepts like "self-esteem" mean nothing to an eight-year-old. Instead, focus on specific, observable phenomena. Not "How's your mood?" but "On a scale of 1-10 with smiley faces, how did you feel at recess today?"

The concept of fairness obsesses school-age children. Everything must be equal, rules must be followed, and violations feel catastrophic. This rigid thinking can manifest in mental health symptoms - the child who melts down when routines change, who cannot tolerate losing games, or who tattles constantly on peers breaking minor rules.

Physical symptoms often mask emotional distress at this age. The stomach aches before school, headaches during math class, vague complaints that disappear on weekends - these somatic symptoms represent genuine distress, not manipulation. The child's emotional pain literally manifests physically because they lack sophisticated emotional vocabulary.

Group therapy shines during school-age years. Children this age desperately want peer acceptance and learn powerfully from each other. Watching another nine-year-old practice deep breathing normalizes coping skills far better than adult instruction. Social skills groups teach pragmatic interaction skills - how to join play, handle disagreements, and read social cues.

Family involvement remains crucial but looks different than in early childhood. School-age children need some autonomy and privacy. The eleven-year-old mortified by their parent's presence during group therapy still needs family support - just delivered more subtly. Teaching parents to support without hovering becomes essential.

Adolescence (Ages 12-18)

Everything changes again with adolescence. Hormones surge, abstract thinking emerges, identity questions dominate, and the push for independence creates constant tension with continued dependency needs. The adolescent brain undergoes massive reconstruction - pruning unused neural connections while myelinating frequently used pathways. It's literally a brain under construction, which explains so much about adolescent behavior.

The prefrontal cortex - responsible for judgment, impulse control, and emotional regulation - won't fully mature until the mid-twenties. Meanwhile, the limbic system (emotional center) develops earlier and operates in overdrive during adolescence. Imagine driving a sports car with a powerful engine but faulty brakes. That's the adolescent brain - intense emotions with limited control mechanisms.

This neurological imbalance creates the perfect storm for risk-taking behavior. The sixteen-year-old who intellectually understands that cutting is dangerous still might use it for emotional regulation. They're not stupid or deliberately self-destructive - their brain literally prioritizes immediate emotional relief over long-term consequences.

Identity formation becomes the primary developmental task. "Who am I?" drives everything. Adolescents try on different identities like clothes - gothic one month, preppy the next. This experimentation is healthy and necessary, though it can alarm adults who want consistency.

Sexual and gender identity questions often emerge during adolescence. The thirteen-year-old questioning their sexuality, the fifteen-year-old exploring gender expression, the seventeen-year-old coming out to family - these identity processes profoundly impact mental health. LGBTQ+ youth face significantly higher mental health risks, not from their identity itself but from society's response to it.

Peer relationships become paramount, often seeming more important than family. This isn't rebellion - it's developmental necessity. Adolescents need to transfer attachment from parents to peers as preparation for adult relationships. The fourteen-year-old who seems to care only about friends' opinions is actually doing important developmental work.

Social media complicates modern adolescent development in unprecedented ways. Today's teenagers navigate identity formation in public digital spaces. Every awkward moment potentially becomes viral content. The pressure for perfection, constant comparison, and 24/7 social availability creates mental health challenges previous generations never faced.

Your therapeutic relationships with adolescents require delicate balance. They need you to treat them as mature individuals while recognizing their continued need for support and structure. Respect their autonomy while maintaining safety boundaries. The fifteen-year-old who insists "I'm not a child!" still needs adult guidance, just delivered respectfully.

Confidentiality becomes complex with adolescents. They need privacy to discuss sensitive topics - substance use, sexual activity, family conflicts. But safety concerns require breaking confidentiality. Navigate this carefully, explaining limits upfront and involving adolescents in safety planning whenever possible.

Abstract thinking abilities allow sophisticated therapy approaches. Adolescents can explore existential questions, examine thinking patterns, and understand complex psychological concepts. Dialectical behavior therapy works well because teenagers can grasp the concept of dialectics - holding two seemingly opposite truths simultaneously.

The push for autonomy creates constant tension. Parents struggle to maintain connection while allowing independence. Adolescents simultaneously want freedom and support. Family therapy during these years often involves negotiating new relationship terms - helping families evolve from parent-child dynamics to something approaching adult relationships.

Neurodevelopmental Considerations

Throughout all developmental stages, neurodevelopmental differences add layers of complexity. Autism spectrum disorder affects social communication and behavior across the lifespan, but manifestations change with development. The autistic four-year-old who lines up toys might become the autistic fourteen-year-old intensely interested in specific topics.

ADHD presents differently across ages too. The hyperactive six-year-old bouncing off walls might become the inattentive sixteen-year-old struggling with executive function. Girls often go undiagnosed because their symptoms - daydreaming, disorganization, emotional dysregulation - don't match stereotypical hyperactive boy presentations.

Learning disabilities impact mental health profoundly. The dyslexic child works twice as hard for half the results, accumulating stress and failure experiences. By adolescence, many develop anxiety or depression secondary to their learning differences. Understanding these connections helps you provide comprehensive care.

Intellectual disabilities require adjusted expectations and interventions. The developmentally delayed twelve-year-old might function emotionally like a six-year-old. Traditional adolescent group therapy won't work - they need interventions matched to developmental, not chronological age.

Twice-exceptional children - those with both gifts and disabilities - face unique challenges. The brilliant child with autism might excel academically while struggling socially. The creative teenager with ADHD might produce amazing art but fail traditional classes. These contrasts create identity confusion and frustration requiring specialized support.

Sensory processing differences affect many children with neurodevelopmental conditions. The child who melts down in noisy environments isn't being difficult - their nervous system literally cannot filter sensory input effectively. Understanding sensory needs helps create supportive environments and prevents behavioral escalations.

Developmental Milestone Tables

Ages 2-3 Years:

- Uses 2-3 word sentences
- Begins parallel play
- Shows defiant behavior ("No!" phase)
- Develops object permanence
- Extreme emotions with little regulation

Ages 4-5 Years:

- Engages in pretend play
- Understands basic emotions (happy, sad, mad, scared)
- Develops initial empathy
- Can follow multi-step directions
- Begins understanding rules

Ages 6-8 Years:

- Concrete logical thinking emerges
- Compares self to peers constantly
- Develops sense of competence/incompetence
- Understands fairness rigidly
- Forms first real friendships

Ages 9-11 Years:

- More sophisticated peer relationships
- Increased independence from family
- Develops personal interests/hobbies
- Beginning body awareness/puberty
- Can understand different perspectives

Ages 12-14 Years:

- Abstract thinking begins
- Identity questioning intensifies
- Peer influence peaks
- Mood swings increase
- Risk-taking behaviors emerge

Ages 15-18 Years:

- Identity consolidation progresses
- Future orientation develops
- Intimate relationships begin
- Independence/dependence conflicts peak
- Existential questions emerge

Brain Development Insights

The brain develops from bottom to top, inside to out. The brainstem (basic survival functions) develops first, then the limbic system (emotions), and finally the cortex (thinking). This sequence explains why young children can walk before they can talk, feel before they can think, and react before they can reflect.

Trauma disrupts typical brain development. When children experience chronic stress, their brains adapt for survival rather than learning. The hypervigilant child constantly scanning for danger can't focus on schoolwork. The dissociative teenager disconnects from their body to escape overwhelming emotions. Understanding trauma's neurological impact guides trauma-informed interventions.

Windows of opportunity exist for different developmental tasks. Language acquisition happens most easily before age seven. Attachment patterns form primarily in the first three years. While brains remain plastic throughout life, these sensitive periods suggest optimal intervention timing.

Family Engagement Strategies Across Development

For Early Childhood:

- Include parents in all treatment sessions
- Teach co-regulation techniques
- Provide parent coaching during interactions
- Focus on attachment strengthening
- Use visual aids for behavior plans

For School-Age:

- Balance child autonomy with parent involvement
- Create separate parent education sessions
- Involve parents in homework/skill practice
- Address parent anxiety about child's struggles
- Foster appropriate independence

For Adolescence:

- Respect teenager's privacy needs
- Offer separate parent support groups
- Negotiate family therapy carefully
- Help parents adjust to changing roles
- Support healthy individuation

The Developmental Lens in Practice

Every interaction requires developmental consideration. The medications dosed differently across ages. The therapy techniques adjusted for cognitive abilities. The family involvement calibrated to developmental needs. The behavioral expectations aligned with brain development.

When a four-year-old can't sit still for a 50-minute therapy session, that's not treatment resistance - it's developmental appropriateness. When a fourteen-year-old refuses family therapy, that's not just oppositional behavior - it's age-appropriate individuation. When an eight-year-old explains their anxiety through stomach aches, that's not manipulation - it's concrete thinking.

Your developmental knowledge transforms generic interventions into developmentally attuned treatment. You don't just teach coping skills - you teach belly breathing to preschoolers, worry boxes to school-agers, and dialectical thinking to teenagers. You don't just assess suicide risk - you understand that young children might not grasp death's permanence while teenagers might hide serious intent.

Practical Applications

Remember that development isn't just linear progression. Stress causes regression - the eleven-year-old who wets the bed during parents' divorce, the teenager who needs stuffed animals during hospitalization. This isn't pathology; it's normal stress response. Meet children where they are developmentally, not where the chart says they should be.

Culture influences developmental expectations too. The independence valued in Western cultures might conflict with collectivist families' interdependence. The "terrible twos" aren't universal - some cultures don't experience this phase because their parenting approaches differ. Always assess development within cultural context.

Individual differences matter enormously. Some children reach milestones early, others late, and both can be perfectly healthy. The anxious parents worried their child isn't talking enough, the teachers concerned about immature behavior - sometimes reassurance about normal variation is the best intervention.

Developmental Understanding

As you continue your journey in pediatric psychiatric nursing, let developmental knowledge inform every interaction. See beyond the diagnosis to the developing person. Recognize that symptoms manifest differently across ages. Understand that interventions must match developmental capacities.

The depressed preschooler, the anxious school-ager, the self-harming teenager - each requires developmentally specific approaches. Your ability to shift between these developmental frameworks, to speak multiple developmental languages, makes you invaluable in pediatric mental health.

This developmental foundation supports everything else you'll learn. Medications work differently in developing brains. Therapies require developmental modifications. Family dynamics shift with developmental stages. Keep this developmental lens at the forefront of your practice, and you'll provide truly developmentally informed care.

Chapter 3: Theoretical Frameworks and Therapeutic Relationships

The teenage boy sits across from you, hoodie pulled up, arms crossed, radiating "leave me alone" energy. He's been on the unit for two days following a suicide attempt, and hasn't spoken more than single syllables to anyone. The treatment team is frustrated. His parents are desperate. Everyone's looking to you, the nurse who spends the most time with him, to somehow break through.

But here's the thing - breaking through isn't about having the perfect words or technique. It's about understanding the theoretical frameworks that guide our interventions and building genuine therapeutic relationships that honor where each young person is developmentally and emotionally. The theories aren't just academic exercises; they're practical tools that shape how you understand behavior, plan interventions, and connect with young people in distress.

Theoretical Foundations That Guide Our Work

The psychodynamic perspective gives us a window into the unconscious processes driving behavior. Now, you won't be conducting psychoanalysis on the unit, but understanding defense mechanisms helps enormously. That teenage boy with his hoodie up? He's using withdrawal as protection. The seven-year-old who becomes the perfect patient, helping with everything? That's reaction formation - managing anxiety by becoming overly compliant.

Children and adolescents often can't articulate their inner conflicts. The ten-year-old doesn't say, "I'm displacing my anger about my parents' divorce onto my teacher." They just start getting in trouble at school. Understanding these unconscious processes helps you see beyond surface behaviors to underlying needs.

Early childhood experiences shape later relationships through what psychodynamic theory calls transference. The teenager who immediately distrusts all male staff might be transferring feelings about an abusive father. The child who desperately seeks approval from every female nurse might be searching for the maternal attention they never received. Recognizing transference helps you understand reactions that seem disproportionate or puzzling.

Your own countertransference matters too. The child who reminds you of your own kid, the teenager whose self-harm triggers your anxiety, the parent whose criticism echoes your own mother's voice - these emotional reactions influence your care. Good pediatric psychiatric nursing requires self-awareness about what each patient evokes in you.

Cognitive-behavioral frameworks revolutionized how we understand and treat mental illness. The core premise - that thoughts, feelings, and behaviors interconnect and influence each other - seems simple but proves powerful. A child thinks "Nobody likes me," feels sad and anxious, then avoids social situations, which prevents making friends, confirming the original thought. Breaking this cycle anywhere can create change.

With younger children, you'll focus more on behavioral interventions since abstract thinking about thoughts hasn't developed. The six-year-old with separation anxiety needs behavioral exposure (gradually increasing separation time) more than cognitive restructuring. You might use sticker charts, reward systems, and structured activities to shape behavior.

By middle school, kids can start recognizing thinking patterns. The anxious eleven-year-old can learn to identify "what if" thoughts and challenge them. "What if I fail the test?" becomes "I've studied and done well before. Even if this test doesn't go perfectly, it won't ruin everything." These cognitive skills become tools they carry forward.

Adolescents can engage in sophisticated CBT work. They can complete thought records, identify cognitive distortions, and run behavioral experiments. The depressed fifteen-year-old who believes "everyone hates me" can test this hypothesis by tracking actual social interactions, often discovering their perception doesn't match reality.

Systems theory reminds us that children don't exist in isolation. They're embedded in multiple systems - family, school, peer groups, community, culture. A child's symptoms often reflect system dysfunction rather than individual pathology. The anxious eight-year-old might be the "identified patient," but the real problem might be parental conflict, family secrets, or systemic stress.

Think about it like this - if you have a fish swimming erratically, you don't just examine the fish. You test the water temperature, check the pH, look for toxins. Similarly, when a child presents with behavioral problems, you assess their entire ecosystem. What's happening at home? How's school going? What's the neighborhood like? What cultural factors influence the family?

Family systems theory introduces concepts like triangulation (child caught between feuding parents), parentification (child taking adult responsibilities), and enmeshment (boundaries too loose between family members). That teenager who seems inexplicably angry? They might be triangulated in their parents' marital problems, forced to choose sides in adult conflicts they shouldn't even know about.

Trauma-informed care has transformed pediatric mental health. We now understand that trauma affects developing brains profoundly. The child exposed to domestic violence, the teenager who experienced sexual abuse, the preschooler who survived multiple foster placements - their brains adapted for survival in dangerous environments.

These adaptations make sense in dangerous contexts but cause problems in safe ones. Hypervigilance helps detect threats but disrupts classroom learning. Dissociation protects from overwhelming emotions but interferes with relationships. Aggression might have prevented victimization but now leads to legal troubles. Understanding behavior through a trauma lens changes everything.

Trauma-informed care means assuming trauma until proven otherwise. Instead of asking "What's wrong with you?" we ask "What happened to you?" This shift from pathology to adaptation, from disorder to response, fundamentally changes how we approach treatment. That aggressive child isn't bad; they're scared. That withdrawn teenager isn't oppositional; they're protecting themselves.

Building Age-Appropriate Therapeutic Relationships

Here's where science becomes art. You can know all the theories, but if you can't connect with a scared five-year-old or a skeptical sixteen-year-old, that knowledge won't help anyone. Therapeutic relationships look different across developmental stages, and your ability to shift your approach accordingly makes all the difference.

With preschoolers, the relationship often builds through play and routine interactions rather than talking. You might spend twenty minutes helping a four-year-old build with blocks before they tell you about the "scary things" at home. Sitting on the floor at their level, using animated expressions, and showing genuine interest in their play builds trust faster than any formal intervention.

Young children need consistency and predictability in relationships. Being the nurse who always has the same special stickers, who remembers their stuffed animal's name, who keeps promises about when you'll return - these small consistencies build enormous trust. For children whose world feels chaotic, your reliability becomes an anchor.

Physical comfort matters at this age too. The preschooler who scrapes their knee needs the band-aid, but more importantly, they need the caring attention that comes with it. Obviously, maintain appropriate boundaries, but don't underestimate the power of permitted safe touch - a high-five, a pat on the back, sitting beside them during a scary procedure.

School-age children need relationships that respect their growing autonomy while providing structure. They want to be included in conversations about their treatment but not overwhelmed with choices. "Would you like to take your medication with juice or water?" offers control without burden. "Do you want to talk about what happened at school, or should we play a game first?" gives them agency in the relationship.

This age group responds well to collaborative approaches. Instead of telling them what to do, involve them in problem-solving. "So when you feel really angry at school, what helps you calm down?" positions them as experts on themselves. When they contribute ideas, they're more likely to follow through.

Humor works wonderfully with school-age kids, but timing matters. The right joke at the right moment can defuse tension and build connection. But forced humor or minimizing their concerns with jokes backfires. Read the room - or rather, read the child.

Adolescent relationships require a delicate dance between treating them as mature individuals and recognizing their continued need for adult support. They have excellent hypocrisy detectors, so authenticity matters more than perfect therapeutic technique. The teenager who asks, "Do you even like this job?" deserves an honest answer, not a deflection.

Respect becomes paramount with adolescents. Knocking before entering their room, asking permission before sharing information with parents (when legally permissible), and acknowledging their perspective even when you disagree - these respectful interactions build credibility. Once you've lost an adolescent's respect, recovering it proves nearly impossible.

Self-disclosure becomes more relevant with teenagers, though boundaries still matter. Sharing that you also struggled with anxiety in high school might build connection. Detailing your entire psychiatric history crosses lines. The key is purposeful, limited disclosure that serves their treatment, not your needs.

Family-Centered Care Approaches

Pediatric psychiatric nursing always involves families, whether they're physically present or notably absent. The family serves as the child's primary context, and lasting change rarely happens without family involvement. But "family-centered" doesn't mean "parent-centered" - it means considering the entire family system's needs and dynamics.

Start by understanding each family's unique structure and culture. The nuclear family with two biological parents represents only one possibility. You'll work with single parents, grandparents raising grandchildren, foster families, adoptive families, chosen families, and everything in between. Each configuration brings strengths and challenges. The grandmother raising her grandson while working two jobs faces different stressors than the two-parent household with resources for private therapy.

Family-centered care means including families as partners, not problems. Yes, family dysfunction often contributes to children's mental health issues. But approaching families as deficient or pathological destroys therapeutic alliance. Instead, assume families are doing their best with available resources and knowledge. Your job is to enhance their capabilities, not replace them.

Communication with families requires constant calibration. Some parents want every detail about their child's treatment. Others feel overwhelmed by too much information. Some families express emotions openly; others maintain stoic facades. Learning each family's communication style and adapting accordingly improves engagement.

The concept of "expressed emotion" helps understand family dynamics' impact on mental health. High expressed emotion - excessive criticism, hostility, or emotional over-involvement - predicts poorer outcomes across psychiatric conditions. But here's the crucial part: high expressed emotion usually stems from love and fear, not malice. The critical parent often fears for their child's future. The over-involved parent desperately wants to prevent suffering.

Working with high expressed emotion families means channeling their intensity productively. Help the critical parent recognize strengths alongside challenges. Teach the over-involved parent that stepping back sometimes helps more than hovering. Frame these changes as more effective ways to help their child, not criticisms of their parenting.

Boundaries between helping and enabling require constant negotiation. The parent who does their teenager's homework isn't helping long-term. The family that walks on eggshells to avoid triggering outbursts inadvertently reinforces the behavior. But changing these patterns feels risky to families already struggling. Your role involves supporting families through the discomfort of change.

Sometimes family involvement means recognizing when families need their own treatment. The depressed parent can't fully support their anxious child. The parents whose marriage is imploding can't provide stable foundation for their acting-out teenager. Referring parents to their own therapy or support services sometimes provides the best pediatric intervention.

Cultural Humility and LGBTQ+ Affirming Care

Cultural competence isn't a destination you reach after reading enough diversity chapters. It's an ongoing journey of cultural humility - recognizing that you'll never fully understand another's cultural experience but committing to continuous learning and adaptation.

Culture influences everything about mental health - how symptoms are expressed, what's considered abnormal, whether help-seeking is acceptable, what interventions feel appropriate. The Latino family might describe anxiety as "nervios" or "susto." The Asian adolescent might express depression through physical symptoms rather than emotional language. The African American family might prefer church counseling over psychiatric treatment.

Rather than assuming you understand someone's culture based on their appearance or last name, ask. "Help me understand how your family views mental health." "What does your community think about medication for emotional problems?" "Are there cultural or religious considerations I should know about?" These questions demonstrate respect and gather essential information.

Language barriers add complexity beyond simple translation. Mental health concepts don't always translate directly. The word "depression" might not exist in someone's primary language. Even with interpreters, nuance gets lost. Whenever possible, provide culturally and linguistically matched providers. When that's impossible, work with professional interpreters familiar with mental health terminology.

Generational differences within immigrant families create unique challenges. The teenager who's become Americanized might clash with parents maintaining traditional values. The child interpreting for parents at appointments holds inappropriate power in the family system. Understanding acculturation stress helps explain some behavioral problems.

LGBTQ+ youth face unique mental health challenges, with significantly higher rates of depression, anxiety, suicidality, and substance use. But here's what's crucial - being LGBTQ+ doesn't cause mental health problems. Minority stress from discrimination, rejection, and internalized negativity creates these disparities.

Creating affirming environments starts with language. Use chosen names and pronouns consistently. If you mess up (and you will), apologize briefly and move on - don't make your mistake about your feelings. Ask about pronouns respectfully: "What pronouns should I use for you?" becomes part of standard intake.

Understand that coming out is a process, not an event. The sixteen-year-old might be out at school but not home, or out to mom but not dad. Respect their decisions about disclosure. Outing someone to their family, even with good intentions, can be dangerous.

Many LGBTQ+ youth face family rejection, ranging from subtle disappointment to complete abandonment. The transgender teenager whose parents use their dead name, the gay adolescent whose family insists it's "just a phase," the bisexual youth told they're "confused" - these experiences compound mental health struggles.

But don't assume all LGBTQ+ youth have unsupportive families. Many families fully embrace their children. The twelve-year-old with two moms might have the most supportive family structure on your unit. Avoid assumptions either way - assess each situation individually.

Putting It All Together

That teenage boy from the beginning? Turns out he'd been struggling with his sexuality for years, terrified of his religious family's reaction. His suicide attempt followed his father finding texts to a boyfriend. Using psychodynamic understanding, you recognize his withdrawal as protection against anticipated rejection. Through a CBT lens, you see how thoughts ("My family will hate me") led to feelings (despair) and behaviors (suicide attempt).

Systems theory helps you understand the family dynamics - religious beliefs, cultural expectations, and genuine love creating an impossible situation. Trauma-informed care recognizes the trauma of anticipated rejection and identity suppression. Cultural humility means understanding his family's religious context without judgment while advocating for his safety and well-being.

Building a therapeutic relationship with him starts small. You mention a band sticker on his notebook, and he actually makes eye contact. You respect his need for space while being consistently available. When he finally starts talking, you listen without immediately trying to fix everything. You validate his pain while instilling hope that things can improve.

Working with his family requires delicate balance. You help them understand that rejection increases suicide risk dramatically while respecting their religious beliefs. You connect them with other religious parents of LGBTQ+ youth who've found acceptance within their faith. You hold space for everyone's pain - the teenager feeling rejected, the parents feeling confused and scared.

Real-World Refinements

Therapeutic relationships don't follow textbook timelines. Some connections happen instantly - the preschooler who immediately trusts you because you remind them of someone safe. Others develop glacially - the traumatized adolescent who tests you for months before risking vulnerability.

Boundaries in pediatric psychiatric nursing require constant attention. The desire to rescue children from difficult situations can overwhelm professional judgment. That foster child you want to adopt, the teenager whose story breaks your heart, the family that reminds you of your own struggles - maintaining therapeutic boundaries while remaining genuinely caring challenges even experienced nurses.

Self-care isn't selfish; it's essential for sustaining therapeutic relationships. Secondary trauma from hearing children's stories, the emotional drain of constant crises, the frustration when systems fail vulnerable youth - these experiences accumulate. Regular supervision, personal therapy, and genuine time away from work help you maintain the emotional availability therapeutic relationships require.

The Healing Power of Relationships

Sometimes the relationship itself is the intervention. The child who's never had a stable adult might need months of consistent interaction before trying any formal therapy. The teenager who's been betrayed by every adult might need to test your limits repeatedly before believing you won't abandon them. The family overwhelmed by their child's diagnosis might need someone to simply witness their struggle before they can engage in treatment.

In pediatric psychiatric nursing, you're not just administering medications or implementing treatment plans. You're offering yourself as a bridge back to trusting relationships. For children whose primary relationships have been sources of pain, your consistent, boundaried, therapeutic presence shows them something different is possible.

Every interaction matters. The way you wake a child for morning medications. How you respond to the teenager's sarcasm. Your reaction when a preschooler has a toileting accident. These moments might seem mundane, but they're building blocks of therapeutic relationships that can literally save lives.

Chapter 4: The Pediatric Psychiatric Assessment

The ten-year-old boy sits in your office chair, swinging his legs that don't quite reach the floor. His mother brought him in because his teacher says he "zones out" in class, his grades are dropping, and he's been complaining of stomach aches every morning before school. But when you ask him directly what's wrong, he shrugs and says "nothing." His mother sighs in frustration. The pediatrician found nothing physically wrong. So here you are, tasked with figuring out what's really going on.

This scenario plays out countless times every day in pediatric mental health settings. Unlike adults who might come seeking help for identified problems, children rarely self-refer. They're brought by worried parents, concerned teachers, or mandated by courts. Your job? To conduct an assessment that's thorough enough to capture the complexity of their struggles, gentle enough to build trust with a scared child, and practical enough to lead to effective treatment.

The pediatric psychiatric assessment isn't just a scaled-down version of an adult assessment. Children's developmental stages, family contexts, and ways of expressing distress require completely different approaches. You're not just assessing the child - you're evaluating an entire ecosystem of relationships, environments, and developmental factors that shape their mental health.

The Biopsychosocial-Spiritual Framework

Think of assessment like being a detective, but instead of solving crimes, you're solving the puzzle of a child's distress. The biopsychosocial-spiritual framework gives you four different lenses through which to examine the situation. Miss any one of these dimensions, and you'll likely miss crucial pieces of the puzzle.

The biological dimension encompasses genetics, neurodevelopment, physical health, and temperament. That anxious eight-year-old? Maybe anxiety runs in the family for three generations. The hyperactive six-year-old might have been born prematurely, affecting brain development. The depressed teenager could have undiagnosed thyroid problems. You're looking at family psychiatric history, prenatal and birth complications, developmental milestones, medical conditions, medications, sleep patterns, appetite, and substance use (yes, even in children).

But here's what makes pediatric assessment different - you can't just ask the child about family psychiatric history. Most kids have no idea that mom takes antidepressants or that uncle Joe was hospitalized for bipolar disorder. You need corroborating information from parents, and sometimes they don't know either. Grandma's "nervous breakdowns" might have been untreated panic disorder. Dad's father who "drank too much" probably had alcohol use disorder plus who knows what else.

The psychological dimension includes cognitive functioning, emotional development, personality traits, coping mechanisms, and trauma history. How does this child understand their world? What are their thoughts about themselves, others, and their future? What defense mechanisms do they use? A seven-year-old might not articulate feeling worthless, but they might draw pictures of themselves as tiny figures overshadowed by everyone else.

Children's psychological functioning must be understood developmentally. The four-year-old who believes monsters live under the bed isn't psychotic - they're demonstrating age-appropriate magical thinking. The eleven-year-old who insists everything must be "fair" isn't showing obsessive traits - they're in the concrete operational stage where rules and fairness become paramount.

The social dimension examines relationships, cultural factors, socioeconomic status, school functioning, peer interactions, and family dynamics. Who are the important people in this child's life? What roles does the child play in different systems? That withdrawn teenager might be the family peacekeeper, managing their parents' marital conflict. The aggressive first-grader might be bullied at school but can't articulate it.

Social assessment in children requires multiple perspectives. The child who teachers describe as "defiant and disruptive" might be described by parents as "sensitive and misunderstood." Neither view is wrong - they're seeing different facets of the same child in different contexts. Your job is to understand why the child presents differently across settings.

The spiritual dimension - often overlooked but incredibly important - includes meaning-making, values, religious or spiritual practices, and existential concerns. Even young children grapple with big questions: Why do bad things happen? What happens when we die? Is there something bigger than us? The nine-year-old whose grandfather just died might be struggling with existential anxiety that manifests as separation anxiety.

Spirituality isn't always religious. It might be the child's connection to nature, their sense of purpose, or what gives their life meaning. The teenager who finds peace in music, the child who feels most themselves when playing sports, the adolescent questioning everything they've been taught - these spiritual dimensions profoundly impact mental health.

Age-Appropriate Clinical Interviews

Here's where the art of pediatric assessment really shines. You can't just sit a five-year-old in a chair and conduct a standard psychiatric interview. Each developmental stage requires different approaches, different questions, and different expectations.

Preschoolers (Ages 3-5) communicate through play more than words. Set up your space with toys, art supplies, and books. Get down on their level - literally. Sit on the floor if needed. Start with something fun and non-threatening. "Wow, I like your shoes! Do they make you run super fast?" Build rapport through play before attempting any formal assessment.

With this age group, observation matters more than verbal report. Watch how they separate from their caregiver. Do they explore your office or cling to mom? How do they play - creatively and flexibly, or rigidly and repetitively? Their play themes reveal inner experiences. The child who makes all the dolls fight might be witnessing domestic violence. The one who puts all the toy animals in jail might feel overly controlled.

Questions for preschoolers must be concrete and simple. Instead of "How do you feel?" try "Is your body feeling good or yucky?" Instead of "Are you anxious?" ask "Does your tummy ever feel funny or hurt when nothing's wrong?" Use visual aids - feeling faces, body outlines to point where they feel things, simple drawings to explain concepts.

School-age children (Ages 6-11) can engage in more direct conversation but still benefit from activities. Have them draw while talking - many children find it easier to discuss difficult topics when their hands are busy. Use worksheets, games, or structured activities to assess different domains. The "worry thermometer" helps quantify anxiety. The "feeling pie chart" explores mixed emotions.

Questions become more sophisticated but remain concrete. "Tell me about the best thing and worst thing that happened this week." "If you had three wishes, what would they be?" "What would your teacher say about you? What would your best friend say?" These questions reveal self-concept, relationships, and concerns without being too direct.

This age group often responds well to normalized, multiple-choice style questions. "Some kids worry about tests, some worry about friends, some worry about their parents. What do you worry about?" This approach reduces shame and makes disclosure easier.

Adolescents (Ages 12-18) can engage in more adult-like interviews but require special consideration of their developmental need for autonomy. Start by explaining confidentiality and its limits clearly. "What we talk about stays between us unless you're unsafe or someone's hurting you." This establishes trust and acknowledges their growing independence.

Begin with less threatening topics - school, friends, interests - before moving to symptoms and concerns. Validate their experiences: "That sounds really frustrating" or "I can see why that would be confusing." Avoid sounding like another lecturing adult. Instead of "You should..." try "What do you think might help?"

Adolescents often minimize or deny problems, especially when parents are present. Always spend some time alone with teenage patients. They might reveal entirely different concerns without parents there - sexual activity, substance use, gender identity questions, family secrets. But respect their privacy boundaries too. Pushing too hard too fast shuts down communication.

Mental Status Exam Modifications

The mental status exam (MSE) provides systematic observation of current functioning, but pediatric versions require significant modifications. You're still assessing the same domains - appearance, behavior, mood, thought process, cognition - but how you assess them changes dramatically with age.

Appearance and behavior observations start the moment the child enters. Is their clothing age-appropriate? Is hygiene adequate? But context matters - the disheveled appearance might reflect poverty, not neglect. The oversized, worn clothes might be hand-me-downs, not indicators of family dysfunction.

Watch for developmental variations in behavior. The fidgety seven-year-old might have ADHD or might just be seven. The teenager slumped in their chair might be depressed or might be performing

45

teenage disdain. Consider cultural norms too - eye contact expectations vary across cultures.

Speech and language assessment must account for developmental norms. The four-year-old who speaks in short sentences isn't necessarily language-delayed. The adolescent using slang you don't understand isn't being disrespectful - they're being an adolescent. Listen for rate, rhythm, volume, and coherence relative to age expectations.

Mood and affect present differently across development. Young children might not label emotions accurately. They might say they're "mad" when they're actually sad or scared. Watch for behavioral indicators - withdrawal might indicate depression, irritability might mask anxiety. Adolescents often present with irritability rather than sadness when depressed.

The range and appropriateness of affect vary developmentally too. Preschoolers normally show rapid mood shifts. School-age children might show restricted affect when uncomfortable. Adolescents might maintain flat affect as a protective stance, not necessarily indicating depression.

Thought process and content assessment requires understanding normal developmental variations. Young children's thoughts jump around - that's normal, not flight of ideas. School-age children might have elaborate fantasies - that's imagination, not psychosis. Adolescents might express dramatic, all-or-nothing thinking - that's developmental, not necessarily pathological.

When assessing for hallucinations, consider developmental factors. Many young children have imaginary friends - totally normal. But if the imaginary friend tells them to hurt themselves or others, that's concerning. Ask about the experience: "Some kids hear voices or see things others don't. Has that ever happened to you?"

Cognitive assessment isn't formal IQ testing but rather general observation of functioning. Can the preschooler follow two-step directions? Does the school-age child seem to understand cause and effect? Can the adolescent think abstractly? Note any significant discrepancies from age expectations.

Attention and concentration vary enormously by age. A five-year-old might focus for 10-15 minutes max. A ten-year-old should sustain attention longer. But context matters - the child who can't focus on your questions might concentrate for hours on video games. That suggests ADHD less than anxiety or oppositional behavior.

Risk Assessment and Safety Planning

This is where pediatric assessment becomes literally life-saving. Suicide is the second leading cause of death in youth aged 10-14. But assessing suicide risk in children requires special considerations beyond adult protocols.

Always ask about suicide directly, using language appropriate to developmental level. With younger children: "Have you ever wished you weren't alive anymore?" or "Have you thought about making yourself not wake up?" With adolescents: "Have you thought about killing yourself?" Being direct doesn't plant ideas - it gives permission to discuss existing thoughts.

Understand that young children might not fully grasp death's permanence. The seven-year-old who says they want to die might think death is reversible, like in video games. Assess their understanding: "What do you think happens when someone dies?" Their answer guides your intervention.

Look for risk factors specific to youth: recent losses, bullying, academic failure, family conflict, questioning sexual orientation or gender identity, access to means (especially firearms in the home), exposure to suicide (including through media), and previous attempts. But also assess protective factors: family support, school connectedness, religious involvement, coping skills, future orientation.

Safety planning with youth must be concrete and practical. Who can they talk to when feeling suicidal? Make a specific list with phone numbers. What activities help them feel better? Create a "coping card" they can carry. Work with parents on means restriction - locking up medications, removing firearms, supervising internet use.

The safety plan must be developmentally appropriate. A young child needs adults to maintain their safety. An adolescent needs some autonomy in their safety plan or they won't use it. Include them in creating it: "What would actually help when you're feeling this way?"

Consider hospitalization criteria carefully. Not every suicidal youth needs inpatient treatment. Factors include: imminence of risk, availability of support, family's ability to maintain safety, child's ability to contract for safety (though never rely solely on contracts), and available outpatient resources.

Assessment Tools and Documentation

Assessment checklists help ensure you don't miss crucial information. Create systematic approaches for different presenting concerns:

Initial Assessment Checklist:

- Chief complaint (child's words and parent's words)
- History of present illness (onset, triggers, course, impact)
- Past psychiatric history (previous treatment, hospitalizations, medications)
- Developmental history (milestones, regressions, concerns)
- Medical history (illnesses, injuries, medications, allergies)
- Family psychiatric history (three generations if possible)
- Social history (living situation, school, friends, activities)
- Trauma history (abuse, neglect, losses, witnessing violence)
- Risk assessment (suicide, self-harm, aggression, victimization)

48

- Protective factors (strengths, supports, interests, goals)

Interview guides structure your assessment while remaining flexible:

Parent Interview Guide:

- "Tell me what brings you here today"
- "When did you first notice these concerns?"
- "What have you tried? What helped? What didn't?"
- "How is this affecting your family?"
- "What are your biggest worries?"
- "What does your child do well?"
- "Tell me about pregnancy and early development"
- "Any family history of mental health or substance issues?"

Child Interview Guide:

- "Do you know why you're here today?"
- "Tell me about your family"
- "What's school like for you?"
- "Who are your friends? What do you do for fun?"
- "What makes you happy? What makes you sad/mad/worried?"
- "If you had a magic wand, what would you change?"
- "Has anyone ever hurt you or touched you in ways that felt wrong?"

Documentation must be thorough yet concise, capturing clinical impressions while remaining objective. Use quotes when possible: The child stated, "I want to die so I can be with grandpa." Describe behaviors specifically: "Child threw three chairs and attempted to bite staff" rather than "Child was aggressive."

Include both symptoms and strengths. Document protective factors as thoroughly as risk factors. Note inconsistencies between reports: "Mother reports daily tantrums; teacher reports no behavioral problems at school." These discrepancies provide valuable clinical information.

Real-World Assessment Challenges

Time constraints plague real-world assessment. You might have 60-90 minutes for an initial evaluation when comprehensive assessment could take hours. Prioritize safety assessment and acute concerns. You can gather additional information over time.

Multiple informants often provide conflicting information. Divorced parents might paint completely different pictures of the same child. Teachers and parents might report opposite behaviors. The child's self-report might match neither. Your job isn't determining who's "right" but understanding why perspectives differ.

Engagement challenges are common. The sullen teenager who won't talk, the hyperactive child who won't sit still, the anxious parent who dominates the conversation - these scenarios require flexibility. Sometimes the best assessment happens while shooting baskets or drawing together, not sitting in chairs.

Cultural considerations profoundly impact assessment. Direct questioning might be considered rude in some cultures. Mental illness might be stigmatized, leading to minimization of symptoms. Religious or spiritual explanations might be offered for psychiatric symptoms. Respect these perspectives while gathering necessary clinical information.

Comorbidity is the rule, not exception in pediatric psychiatry. The child with ADHD likely also has learning disabilities, anxiety, or oppositional behaviors. The depressed teenager might also struggle with eating disorders, substance use, or self-harm. Comprehensive assessment catches comorbidities that might otherwise be missed.

Pulling It All Together

That ten-year-old from the beginning? Through careful assessment, you discover he's been bullied at school for months but was too ashamed to tell anyone. His "zoning out" is dissociation from overwhelming anxiety. The stomach aches are somatic symptoms. His parents' recent separation, which they thought they'd hidden well, has destabilized his sense of safety.

Using the biopsychosocial-spiritual framework, you identify biological vulnerabilities (family history of anxiety), psychological factors (tendency toward internalization), social stressors (bullying, family changes), and spiritual concerns (questioning why bad things happen to good people). Your developmentally appropriate interview helped him finally share his secret through drawing and play. The mental status exam revealed anxiety symptoms masked as attention problems. Risk assessment showed no current suicidality but identified warning signs to monitor.

This thorough assessment guides treatment planning. You'll need interventions addressing the bullying, family therapy for the separation adjustment, CBT for anxiety, possible medication evaluation, and school consultation. Without comprehensive assessment, he might have been misdiagnosed with ADHD and given stimulants that would worsen his anxiety.

Essential Takeaways for Practice

Assessment sets the foundation for everything that follows. Rush through it, and you'll miss crucial information that derails treatment. Take time to build rapport, gather multiple perspectives, and understand the child within their developmental and environmental context.

Always assess through developmental lens. What's normal at five looks like pathology at fifteen. What's concerning in one culture might be typical in another. Stay curious, humble, and willing to revise your impressions as you learn more.

Safety always comes first. Never skip risk assessment, even when it feels awkward or time pressures mount. The child who seems least likely to be at risk might be hiding the most pain. Ask directly, plan carefully, and document thoroughly.

The best assessment tool is relationship. All the checklists and screening instruments can't replace genuine connection with a child and family. When they trust you enough to share their truth, that's when real assessment happens.

Chapter 5: Evidence-Based Screening and Assessment Tools

You're working the afternoon shift when a mother arrives with her three-year-old daughter. "Something's not right," she insists, though the pediatrician found nothing wrong. The child seems typical at first glance - playing quietly, making occasional eye contact. But mom describes behaviors that concern her: lining up toys obsessively, meltdowns over routine changes, echolalia. Do you dismiss parent concerns? Order extensive testing? Or do you have systematic ways to assess what's really happening?

This scenario highlights why standardized screening tools have become indispensable in pediatric mental health. Gone are the days of relying solely on clinical intuition. Today's evidence-based practice demands objective measures that can detect problems early, track progress over time, and ensure we're not missing subtle but significant symptoms. But with hundreds of available tools, how do you choose the right one? How do you administer them appropriately across different ages? And most importantly, how do you integrate screening results with clinical judgment to guide treatment?

Early Childhood Tools (Ages 2-5)

The early years present unique assessment challenges. Young children can't complete self-report measures. Their behavior varies dramatically across settings. Normal development includes wide variation. Yet early identification and intervention can literally change life trajectories. That's why having the right tools matters so much.

The ASQ-3 (Ages & Stages Questionnaires, Third Edition) serves as a first-line developmental screening tool. Parents complete

30 questions about their child's abilities in five domains: communication, gross motor, fine motor, problem-solving, and personal-social. What makes the ASQ-3 brilliant is its simplicity. Questions are concrete and observable: "Does your child walk up stairs by himself?" "Can she tell you her first and last name?"

The ASQ-3 takes about 10-15 minutes for parents to complete and 2-3 minutes for you to score. Scores fall into three zones: above cutoff (on track), close to cutoff (provide activities and rescreen), or below cutoff (refer for evaluation). But here's what the manual doesn't emphasize enough - parental concern matters even when scores look fine. If a parent says something feels wrong despite normal ASQ-3 scores, keep investigating.

The M-CHAT-R/F (Modified Checklist for Autism in Toddlers-Revised with Follow-up) specifically screens for autism spectrum disorder between 16-30 months. Twenty questions assess social communication and repetitive behaviors. "If you point at something across the room, does your child look at it?" "Does your child play pretend or make-believe?"

What makes the M-CHAT-R/F powerful is its two-stage process. The initial parent questionnaire identifies risk. Then the follow-up interview clarifies failed items, reducing false positives. A child might fail "Does your child point to show you something interesting?" But follow-up reveals they bring objects to show you instead - culturally different but functionally equivalent communication.

Scoring seems straightforward - fail two or more critical items or three total items triggers follow-up. But interpretation requires nuance. Some children fail items due to developmental delays, not autism. Others pass the M-CHAT-R/F but still have autism - especially girls and children without intellectual disabilities who often present subtly.

PEARLS (Pediatric ACEs and Related Life-Events Screener) addresses trauma and adversity in young children. Unlike the original ACEs questionnaire that asks adults about childhood retrospectively, PEARLS captures current childhood experiences. Items include traditional ACEs (abuse, neglect, household dysfunction) plus additional stressors like discrimination, neighborhood violence, and deportation fears.

The power of PEARLS lies in opening conversations about topics parents might not volunteer. That mother who seems perfectly put-together might be fleeing domestic violence. The family that appears stable might be facing eviction. These stressors profoundly impact child development and behavior, but without systematic screening, they often remain hidden.

But PEARLS requires careful administration. Never hand parents the questionnaire cold - explain its purpose, normalize that many families face challenges, and ensure privacy. Have resources ready. If a parent endorses current domestic violence, you need immediate safety planning, not just a referral.

Additional early childhood tools serve specific purposes. The CBCL/1.5-5 (Child Behavior Checklist) provides comprehensive behavioral assessment. The PSC-17 (Pediatric Symptom Checklist) offers brief general screening. The SCARED-P (parent version) assesses anxiety symptoms. Each tool has strengths and limitations you need to understand.

The key with early childhood screening is multimethod, multi-informant assessment. Parents see behaviors at home. Teachers observe peer interactions. You witness parent-child dynamics. Standardized tools provide systematic data collection, but they complement rather than replace clinical observation.

School-Age Instruments (Ages 6-11)

School-age children can begin participating in their own assessment, though parent and teacher reports remain crucial. This developmental period allows for more sophisticated screening but requires careful consideration of cognitive and reading abilities.

The PSC (Pediatric Symptom Checklist) comes in two versions - parent-report (PSC-35) and youth self-report (Y-PSC-35 for ages 11+). Thirty-five items screen for psychosocial problems across internalizing, externalizing, and attention domains. "Complains of aches and pains," "Fights with others," "Has trouble concentrating" - simple statements rated never/sometimes/often.

What makes the PSC valuable is its brevity and breadth. In five minutes, you screen for multiple problem areas. Scores above cutoffs suggest need for further evaluation, not specific diagnoses. The child who scores high on attention items needs comprehensive ADHD assessment, not immediate medication.

The PSC works in various settings - primary care, schools, mental health clinics. But context affects interpretation. Elevated scores in medical settings might reflect adjustment to illness rather than psychiatric disorders. Cultural factors influence scores too - some cultures report more somatic symptoms, others minimize emotional expressions.

The SCARED (Screen for Child Anxiety Related Disorders) specifically assesses anxiety symptoms. Forty-one items map onto anxiety disorders: separation anxiety, generalized anxiety, panic, social anxiety, and school avoidance. Both child and parent versions exist, often revealing interesting discrepancies.

Children might report internal anxiety parents don't observe. "I worry about people liking me" might score high on child-report but low on parent-report. Conversely, parents might notice avoidance behaviors children don't acknowledge. These discrepancies aren't problems to resolve but valuable clinical information about different perspectives.

SCARED scores above 25 suggest significant anxiety warranting further evaluation. But subscale scores matter too. The child with elevated social anxiety scores needs different interventions than one with separation anxiety. Use the SCARED to guide, not make, diagnostic decisions.

The Vanderbilt Assessment Scales comprehensively evaluate ADHD and comorbid conditions. Parent and teacher versions include symptom ratings plus impairment measures. Beyond ADHD symptoms, they screen for oppositional defiant disorder, conduct disorder, anxiety, and depression.

What sets Vanderbilt apart is its emphasis on functional impairment. A child might have ADHD symptoms but function well with environmental supports. Another might have fewer symptoms but significant impairment. Treatment decisions should consider both symptomatology and functioning.

The Vanderbilt requires both parent and teacher reports for accurate assessment. Teachers observe attention and behavior in structured settings with peer comparisons. Parents see homework struggles, morning routines, and social challenges. Discrepancies between settings provide diagnostic clues - ADHD symptoms should appear across settings, while anxiety might manifest primarily at school.

School-age screening challenges include reading levels, response bias, and developmental variation. Some eight-year-olds read at third-grade level, others at first-grade. Always ensure children understand questions. Read items aloud if needed. Watch for response patterns suggesting random answering or trying to please.

Kids this age might not recognize symptoms as problems. The anxious child might think everyone worries constantly. The depressed child might believe they deserve to feel bad. Normalizing statements help: "Some kids feel this way, some don't. How about you?"

Adolescent Screening (Ages 12-18)

Adolescent screening introduces new complexities. Teens can complete sophisticated self-report measures but might minimize or exaggerate symptoms. Confidentiality becomes paramount. Risk behaviors require assessment. Identity and relationship issues emerge.

The PHQ-9A (Patient Health Questionnaire-9 for Adolescents) screens for depression with modifications for youth. Nine items assess DSM criteria for major depression, plus questions about functional impairment. The adolescent version adds questions about suicide specific to teens.

Scores of 10+ suggest moderate depression warranting treatment. But individual items matter too. Any positive response to suicide questions requires immediate assessment, regardless of total score. The teen who scores 8 but endorses suicide ideation needs more urgent intervention than one scoring 15 without suicidality.

The PHQ-9A's brevity enables repeated administration to track treatment response. Scores should decrease with effective treatment. If not, reconsider diagnosis or treatment approach. Maybe it's bipolar disorder, not unipolar depression. Maybe medication isn't working. Maybe environmental stressors overwhelm treatment effects.

The Columbia Suicide Severity Rating Scale (C-SSRS) provides systematic suicide risk assessment. Unlike simple yes/no suicide questions, the C-SSRS distinguishes wish to die, suicidal ideation, intent, plan, and attempts. This granularity guides intervention intensity.

The teen who says "Sometimes I wish I wouldn't wake up" needs different intervention than one with specific plan and intent. The C-SSRS helps determine level of care - outpatient therapy, intensive outpatient, partial hospitalization, or inpatient treatment.

But the C-SSRS is just one tool in suicide assessment. Clinical judgment, protective factors, and support systems matter equally. The teen with passive ideation but strong family support might be safer than one with vague ideation but multiple risk factors and isolation.

The CRAFFT screens for substance use in adolescents. Six questions create the acronym: Car (riding with intoxicated driver),

58

Relax (using to relax), Alone (using alone), Forget (blackouts), Friends/Family (others suggesting cutting down), Trouble (trouble from using).

Two or more positive responses suggest problematic use warranting further assessment. But even one positive deserves attention. The teen who uses alone shows different risk than social users. The CRAFFT opens conversation about substance use without extensive interrogation.

Cultural considerations affect CRAFFT interpretation. In some communities, substance use is normalized. In others, any use brings severe consequences. Understanding context helps you intervene appropriately - harm reduction for some, abstinence for others.

The GAD-7 (Generalized Anxiety Disorder-7) efficiently screens for anxiety. Seven items assess worry and physical symptoms. Scores of 10+ suggest clinically significant anxiety. Like the PHQ-9A, it's brief enough for repeated administration to track treatment.

But adolescent anxiety often presents as irritability, not worry. The teen snapping at everyone might be anxious, not oppositional. The GAD-7 might miss anxiety presenting as somatic complaints, school refusal, or substance use. Use it as one piece of comprehensive assessment.

Specialized Assessments

Beyond general screening, specialized tools assess specific populations, symptoms, or circumstances. Knowing when and how to use these tools enhances assessment precision.

Trauma assessment requires developmentally appropriate tools. The UCLA PTSD Reaction Index assesses trauma exposure and symptoms across ages. The Trauma Symptom Checklist for Children captures various trauma responses. The Child Dissociative Checklist screens for dissociation often missed in standard assessment.

But trauma assessment demands special care. Detailed trauma inquiry can be retraumatizing. Some children need stabilization before trauma processing. Others aren't ready to disclose. Trauma screening opens doors but doesn't require walking through them immediately.

Cognitive screening helps identify intellectual disabilities or giftedness affecting presentation. The Kaufman Brief Intelligence Test provides quick cognitive assessment. Academic achievement tests identify learning disabilities. Executive function rating scales assess organizational and planning abilities.

Cognitive factors profoundly impact mental health treatment. The child with intellectual disability needs concrete, simplified interventions. The gifted child might need existential discussions beyond their years. Learning disabilities create secondary mental health problems through repeated failure experiences.

Cultural assessment tools help understand symptoms within cultural context. The Cultural Formulation Interview explores cultural identity, conceptualization of distress, and treatment preferences. The ADDRESSING framework systematically assesses multiple cultural factors: Age, Developmental and acquired Disabilities, Religion, Ethnicity, Socioeconomic status, Sexual orientation, Indigenous heritage, National origin, and Gender.

But cultural assessment can't be reduced to checklists. It requires genuine curiosity, humility, and recognition that culture influences everything - symptom expression, help-seeking, treatment engagement, and recovery concepts.

Tool Selection Strategies

With hundreds of available tools, selection becomes crucial. Here's a practical framework:

Start with purpose. Are you screening broadly or assessing specific concerns? Initial evaluations benefit from broad screeners (PSC,

SDQ). Follow-up assessments need targeted tools (PHQ-9A for depression, SCARED for anxiety).

Consider developmental stage. Preschoolers need parent-report measures. School-age children can contribute but need simple language. Adolescents complete sophisticated self-reports but might minimize symptoms.

Match reading level. Many tools require sixth-grade reading level or higher. Assess literacy before handing out forms. Read items aloud if needed. Use pictorial scales for younger or lower-literacy populations.

Account for time constraints. Primary care settings need ultra-brief screeners. Comprehensive evaluations allow longer batteries. But more isn't always better - assessment fatigue reduces validity.

Think about repeated administration. If tracking treatment response, choose tools designed for repetition. The PHQ-9A and GAD-7 work well weekly. The CBCL is too long for frequent use.

Ensure cultural validity. Tools developed on white, middle-class samples might not apply universally. Check whether translations are validated, not just translated. Understand cultural factors affecting scores.

Digital Platforms and Innovation

Technology is revolutionizing assessment administration and interpretation. Digital platforms offer advantages but require thoughtful implementation.

Electronic administration through tablets or computers offers several benefits. Automatic scoring reduces errors. Skip patterns ensure appropriate questions. Data immediately enters electronic records. Kids often prefer tablets to paper forms.

But technology creates barriers too. Not all families have digital literacy. Screen time might already be problematic. Technical glitches disrupt assessment flow. Always have paper backups available.

Adaptive testing adjusts question difficulty based on responses. This reduces assessment length while maintaining precision. Computer algorithms select optimal items for each individual. But adaptive testing requires sophisticated platforms many settings lack.

Ecological momentary assessment captures symptoms in real-time through smartphone apps. Teens rate mood multiple times daily, revealing patterns invisible in retrospective reports. But compliance varies, and constant symptom monitoring might increase rumination.

Artificial intelligence increasingly aids interpretation. Algorithms identify response patterns suggesting invalid responding. Machine learning predicts treatment response based on assessment profiles. But AI supplements, never replaces, clinical judgment.

Integration with Clinical Practice

Assessment tools provide data, not answers. Integration with clinical judgment, observation, and context creates meaningful understanding.

Scores are starting points, not endpoints. The child who scores below SCARED cutoffs but describes clear anxiety needs treatment. The adolescent with elevated PHQ-9A scores might be responding to acute stressor, not experiencing major depression. Use scores to guide further inquiry.

Multiple informants provide perspective. When parent and child reports differ dramatically, explore why. Maybe parents don't know about bullying. Maybe children don't recognize their irritability affects others. Discrepancies reveal important dynamics.

Change scores matter more than absolute scores. The child whose SCARED score drops from 35 to 25 shows improvement despite remaining above cutoff. The teen whose PHQ-9A increases from 8 to 12 needs intervention adjustment despite staying in "mild" range.

Context determines interpretation. Elevated scores during divorce proceedings might reflect adjustment, not disorder. High anxiety before starting new school might be adaptive. Consider timing, stressors, and developmental factors.

Practical Implementation Guide

Here's how to build assessment into real-world practice:

Create assessment protocols for common presentations. Depression protocol: PHQ-9A, C-SSRS, functional assessment. ADHD protocol: Vanderbilt parent and teacher, executive function ratings, academic screening. Having protocols ensures consistency and thoroughness.

Train staff appropriately. Everyone administering tools needs training. Receptionists handing out screeners need basic understanding. Nurses scoring measures need interpretation knowledge. Providers need advanced training in integration and clinical decision-making.

Build feedback loops. Share results with families immediately. "Your responses suggest significant anxiety. Let's talk about what that means and how we can help." Feedback engages families and validates their concerns.

Document thoughtfully. Record not just scores but interpretation. "PHQ-9A = 18 suggesting moderate-severe depression. Items 3 and 4 elevated indicating sleep disturbance. Suicide item negative. Plan: CBT-I for sleep, monitor mood."

Re-assess regularly. Initial assessment establishes baseline. Repeated assessment tracks progress. Don't wait until treatment ends - regular monitoring allows timely adjustments.

Moving Forward

That three-year-old from the opening? The M-CHAT-R/F identified several red flags. Follow-up clarified some concerns but confirmed others. Combined with clinical observation and developmental assessment, early autism spectrum disorder was identified. Early intervention started immediately, potentially changing her developmental trajectory.

Evidence-based screening tools don't replace clinical skills - they enhance them. They ensure we ask the right questions, catch problems we might miss, and track whether our interventions actually work. Used thoughtfully, they transform hunches into data, concerns into action plans, and assessment into effective treatment.

Chapter 6: Diagnostic Formulation and Treatment Planning

The team meeting feels tense. You're discussing a thirteen-year-old who's been on the unit for a week. The psychiatrist sees clear ADHD. The therapist insists it's trauma-related. The teacher consultant mentions possible learning disabilities. The family therapist notes significant family dysfunction. Everyone's right, and everyone's missing the bigger picture. How do you integrate these perspectives into a coherent understanding that actually helps this child?

This scenario repeats daily in pediatric mental health settings. Children rarely present with single, clear-cut diagnoses. Instead, they arrive with complex combinations of symptoms, circumstances, and developmental factors that defy simple categorization. Your ability to synthesize information into meaningful diagnostic formulations and practical treatment plans determines whether that child gets better or continues struggling despite everyone's best efforts.

DSM-5-TR Pediatric Adaptations

The DSM-5-TR provides our diagnostic framework, but using it with children requires understanding its developmental adaptations and limitations. Adult criteria don't always translate directly to pediatric populations. A five-year-old's depression looks nothing like an adult's. An anxious eight-year-old might present with anger, not worry. Adolescent mania might manifest as extreme irritability rather than euphoria.

Neurodevelopmental disorders received major updates recognizing that these conditions begin in childhood. Autism spectrum disorder now encompasses what used to be separate diagnoses, acknowledging the spectrum nature of presentation. The intellectually disabled teenager with few words and the highly verbal child with social communication challenges both fall within ASD, requiring vastly different interventions.

ADHD criteria now explicitly state symptoms must be present before age twelve, not seven, recognizing that inattentive type often isn't identified until academic demands increase. The DSM-5-TR also allows ADHD diagnosis alongside ASD, acknowledging these frequently co-occur. This change dramatically impacts treatment - the child with both conditions needs interventions addressing both attention and social communication.

Disruptive mood dysregulation disorder (DMDD) was created specifically for children with severe irritability and frequent temper outbursts. Before DMDD, these kids often received bipolar diagnoses, leading to inappropriate mood stabilizer treatment. DMDD recognizes that chronic irritability in children usually isn't bipolar disorder but requires its own understanding and intervention approach.

The criteria are strict - temper outbursts three or more times weekly, persistent irritability between outbursts, symptoms for twelve or more months, onset before age ten. This prevents overdiagnosis while capturing genuinely impaired children. But here's what's tricky - DMDD can't coexist with oppositional defiant disorder, intermittent explosive disorder, or bipolar disorder. If criteria for multiple disorders are met, diagnostic hierarchy rules apply.

Anxiety disorders show important pediatric modifications. Separation anxiety disorder, while possible in adults, primarily affects children. The six-year-old who can't sleep alone, the ten-year-old with school refusal, the teenager who texts mom constantly - these behaviors might reflect developmentally inappropriate separation anxiety.

Selective mutism, almost exclusively beginning in childhood, is now classified as an anxiety disorder rather than "other" category. This shift recognizes that children who don't speak in certain settings aren't being oppositional - they're experiencing anxiety so severe it literally steals their voice.

Trauma and stressor-related disorders include important developmental considerations. PTSD criteria for children six and younger differ from older children and adults. Young children might show trauma through play reenactment rather than intrusive memories. They might display behavioral regression rather than emotional numbing.

Reactive attachment disorder and disinhibited social engagement disorder specifically address severe neglect in early childhood. These diagnoses require evidence of pathogenic care - not just inadequate parenting but extreme neglect or multiple placement changes. They're serious diagnoses with long-term implications, not labels for difficult behavior.

Key developmental considerations run throughout DSM-5-TR. Many disorders specify symptom differences across ages. Major depression might manifest as irritability rather than sadness in children. Social anxiety might present as tantrums rather than avoidance in preschoolers. Substance use disorders have different criteria for adolescents than adults, recognizing developmental differences in tolerance and withdrawal.

But the DSM-5-TR has limitations in pediatric populations. It doesn't adequately address subsyndromal presentations common in developing children. The anxious child who doesn't quite meet criteria for any specific anxiety disorder still needs treatment. Dimensional approaches considering symptom severity sometimes serve children better than categorical diagnoses.

Case Formulation Models

Diagnosis tells you what. Formulation tells you why and how. It's the difference between knowing a child has ADHD and understanding how their ADHD interacts with learning disabilities, family chaos, and social rejection to create their unique presentation.

The "4 Ps" model provides a practical framework: Predisposing, Precipitating, Perpetuating, and Protective factors.

Predisposing factors are vulnerabilities present before symptom onset. Genetic loading for mental illness, difficult temperament, early trauma, prenatal exposures - these set the stage for later problems. The child with family history of anxiety and behaviorally inhibited temperament has heightened risk for anxiety disorders.

Precipitating factors trigger symptom emergence. Parents' divorce, bullying onset, academic failure, puberty - these events activate vulnerabilities. The genetically vulnerable child might develop depression after their first romantic rejection. Understanding precipitants helps predict future triggers.

Perpetuating factors maintain symptoms once started. Avoidance maintains anxiety. Social withdrawal worsens depression. Negative attention reinforces disruptive behavior. Family accommodation prevents exposure to feared situations. Identifying perpetuating factors reveals intervention targets.

Protective factors buffer against symptoms or promote resilience. Strong attachment to one caregiver, academic success, special talents, cultural identity, religious involvement - these factors support recovery. Building on protective factors often works better than just reducing risk factors.

The biopsychosocial formulation integrates multiple levels of understanding:

Biological factors: "This 10-year-old has genetic vulnerability to ADHD (father diagnosed), prenatal nicotine exposure, and chronic sleep deprivation from sleep apnea. These biological factors impair attention regulation and emotional control."

Psychological factors: "Repeated academic failures led to learned helplessness and negative self-concept. He copes through class clown behavior, gaining peer attention while avoiding academic demands. Concrete operational thinking limits his ability to understand long-term consequences."

Social factors: "Chaotic home environment with inconsistent discipline makes symptom management difficult. Teacher's punitive approach exacerbates oppositional behavior. Peer rejection following aggressive incidents reduces social support."

This integrated formulation guides multilevel intervention - medication for ADHD, sleep study for apnea, cognitive-behavioral therapy for self-concept, parent training for home structure, teacher consultation for classroom management, social skills training for peer relationships.

Developmental formulation considers how the child's developmental stage influences their presentation and needs:

"This 7-year-old's anxiety symptoms must be understood within concrete operational thinking. She cannot yet think abstractly about probability, so cognitive restructuring won't work. Her need for predictability and rules reflects normal developmental needs amplified by anxiety. Intervention must be behaviorally focused with heavy parent involvement, as she lacks emotional regulation skills for independent coping."

Compare this to an adolescent formulation:

"This 16-year-old's depression occurs during identity formation stage. Academic pressure threatens her developing sense of competence. Social comparison through social media amplifies negative self-evaluation. Her abstract thinking enables rumination but also allows for cognitive therapy. Treatment must respect her developmental need for autonomy while maintaining safety."

Cultural formulation examines how culture shapes symptom expression, understanding, and treatment preferences:

"This Latino adolescent's distress presents somatically ('nervios') rather than psychological symptoms, consistent with cultural expression patterns. Family's religious attribution of symptoms as spiritual trial affects treatment engagement. Collective family orientation means individual therapy feels culturally dystonic. Strong extended family provides support but also pressure. Incorporating culturally syntonic interventions like family therapy and possibly consulting with religious leader may improve engagement."

Collaborative Treatment Planning

Treatment planning isn't something you do *to* families but *with* them. Collaborative planning increases engagement, improves outcomes, and respects family autonomy. But collaboration with children and adolescents requires developmental consideration.

Engaging children in treatment planning looks different across ages. Preschoolers can't set treatment goals, but they can choose reward stickers. School-age children can identify what they want to change: "I want to worry less about tests." Adolescents can actively participate in goal-setting and intervention selection.

Use developmentally appropriate language. Instead of "We'll work on emotional regulation," try "We'll help you handle big feelings better." Instead of "cognitive restructuring," say "We'll practice thinking in ways that help you feel better."

Make abstract concepts concrete. Use feelings thermometers, worry scales, or behavior charts. The eight-year-old who can't describe anxiety verbally can point to where their worry thermometer is today. Visual representations help children understand their progress.

Parent engagement requires balancing multiple roles. Parents are historians providing background, co-clients needing support, and co-therapists implementing interventions. Understanding which role is primary at any moment guides your approach.

Some parents want to fix everything immediately. Others feel overwhelmed and helpless. Some blame themselves; others blame the child. Meeting parents where they are emotionally helps build alliance. "This is really hard. You're doing your best in a tough situation" validates their struggle while encouraging engagement.

Address parent concerns directly. If they fear medication will change their child's personality, discuss this openly. If they worry about stigma, problem-solve discretely. Unaddressed concerns lead to non-adherence or dropout.

SMART Goals Development

SMART goals - Specific, Measurable, Achievable, Relevant, Time-bound - transform vague wishes into actionable plans. But creating SMART goals with children requires creativity and flexibility.

Specific means clearly defined behaviors or symptoms. "Be good" isn't specific. "Follow morning routine without reminders" is specific. "Feel better" isn't specific. "Reduce panic attacks from daily to weekly" is specific.

With younger children, make goals concrete and observable. "Use words instead of hitting when angry" rather than "improve emotional regulation." Picture cards showing goal behaviors help young children understand expectations.

Measurable means you can track progress objectively. "Improve mood" isn't measurable. "Increase pleasant activities from zero to three weekly" is measurable. "Better focus" isn't measurable. "Complete homework 4 out of 5 days" is measurable.

Use child-friendly measurement. Sticker charts, point systems, or apps can track behaviors. Mood rating scales with faces help children self-monitor. The key is making measurement part of routine, not burden.

Achievable means realistic given the child's capabilities and circumstances. The severely depressed teen won't suddenly become social butterfly. The child with severe ADHD won't immediately sit still for hours. Set goals that stretch but don't break.

Start with small wins to build momentum. If the school-refusing child hasn't attended in months, the first goal might be driving to school parking lot, not full attendance. Success breeds motivation for bigger challenges.

Relevant means meaningful to the child and family. Goals imposed without buy-in fail. The teenager who doesn't see anxiety as problematic won't engage in exposure therapy. Find what matters to them - maybe social anxiety prevents dating or driving.

Connect goals to child's interests. The Minecraft-obsessed child might track mood using Minecraft characters. The athlete might frame anxiety management as mental training for sports performance.

Time-bound means having deadlines that create urgency without overwhelming. "Someday" never comes. "By next Tuesday" creates accountability. But timelines must be realistic - symptom reduction takes time.

Use natural timeframes when possible. School quarters, sports seasons, or holidays provide built-in checkpoints. "Before basketball season starts" feels more meaningful than arbitrary dates.

Level of Care Determination

Determining appropriate care level - outpatient, intensive outpatient, partial hospitalization, residential, or inpatient - requires careful assessment of severity, safety, and support systems.

Outpatient treatment works for stable children with supportive families. Weekly therapy and monthly medication management suffice when symptoms are mild-moderate, safety risk is low, and families can maintain structure. Most children receive outpatient care successfully.

But outpatient requires certain capabilities. Families must transport children consistently. Children need basic safety even between sessions. If parents can't implement behavior plans or ensure medication compliance, outpatient won't work regardless of symptom severity.

Intensive outpatient (IOP) provides more support without removing children from home. Three to five sessions weekly might include individual therapy, group therapy, and family therapy. IOP works well for moderate symptoms requiring more than weekly contact but not constant supervision.

School-based IOP programs minimize disruption while providing intensive support. After-school programs allow academic continuity. Summer IOPs provide structure during high-risk unstructured time.

Partial hospitalization (PHP) provides day treatment with evenings at home. Children attend five days weekly for six to eight hours, receiving therapy, medication management, school support, and therapeutic milieu. PHP serves as step-down from inpatient or step-up from outpatient.

PHP works when children need daily support but have safe home environments. The suicidal teen with supportive parents might attend PHP daily while sleeping at home. This maintains family connections while providing intensive treatment.

Residential treatment provides 24-hour care in non-hospital settings for weeks to months. Children with severe, persistent symptoms not responding to community treatment might need residential care. Complex trauma, severe behavioral problems, or family inability to maintain safety might indicate residential placement.

But residential treatment disrupts everything - family relationships, friendships, school continuity. It should be last resort after exhausting community options. The goal is stabilization and skill-building for successful community return.

Inpatient psychiatric hospitalization provides acute stabilization for imminent safety risks. The actively suicidal child, the psychotic adolescent, the violent youth endangering others - these situations require inpatient care. But hospitalization is brief crisis intervention, not definitive treatment.

Average pediatric psychiatric admission lasts 5-10 days - enough for safety stabilization and medication initiation, not personality restructuring. Discharge planning starts at admission, arranging follow-up before crisis resolution glow fades.

Treatment Matching and Sequencing

Not all interventions work for all conditions or all children. Treatment matching considers diagnosis, development, family factors, and practical constraints.

Evidence-based treatments have research support for specific conditions. CBT for adolescent depression, parent management training for oppositional behavior, exposure therapy for anxiety - these aren't interchangeable. Using DBT for simple phobia wastes resources. Using play therapy for severe OCD delays effective treatment.

But "evidence-based" doesn't mean rigid manualization. Adapt interventions for individual children. The CBT protocol designed for typically developing adolescents needs modification for intellectually disabled youth. Cultural adaptations improve engagement for minority families.

Treatment sequencing matters when children have multiple problems. Do you treat ADHD or anxiety first? Depression or substance use? Sometimes one problem maintains others - treating ADHD might resolve secondary oppositional behavior. Sometimes problems interact - anxiety and depression might need simultaneous treatment.

Consider developmental windows. The preschooler with autism needs early intensive behavioral intervention now - social anxiety can wait. The suicidal teenager needs immediate safety stabilization before addressing learning disabilities.

Combined treatments often work better than single interventions. ADHD responds best to medication plus behavioral intervention. Adolescent depression improves more with therapy plus medication than either alone. But more isn't always better - too many simultaneous interventions overwhelm families.

Documentation and Communication

Your treatment plan is only as good as its documentation and communication. Clear, specific plans guide treatment and satisfy regulatory requirements.

Problem lists should be specific and prioritized. Not just "depression" but "Major Depressive Disorder, moderate, with anxious distress, onset 6 months ago following parents' divorce." Not just "behavioral problems" but "Oppositional Defiant Disorder, severe, primarily in home setting, with aggressive features."

Prioritize by severity, impairment, and family concerns. The child with mild ADHD and severe anxiety might need anxiety treatment first. But if family primarily seeks help for school failure from ADHD, starting there builds alliance.

Intervention descriptions must be specific enough for implementation. "Family therapy" doesn't provide guidance. "Weekly structural family therapy focused on establishing clear hierarchy, consistent limits, and positive parent-child interactions" tells everyone what to expect.

Include frequency, duration, and responsible parties. "CBT for depression, 12 weekly 50-minute sessions with Dr. Smith, homework reviewed by parents between sessions" creates accountability.

Outcome measures should link to goals. If the goal is reducing anxiety, specify how you'll measure - SCARED scores, number of panic attacks, school attendance rates. Plan reassessment intervals - monthly medication checks, quarterly treatment plan reviews.

Crisis planning belongs in every treatment plan. What are warning signs? Who does family call? What coping strategies help? Having written crisis plans prevents panicked decision-making during actual crises.

Real-World Challenges and Solutions

Diagnostic uncertainty is common in pediatrics. The seven-year-old with attention problems might have ADHD, anxiety, trauma effects, or typical development. Sometimes you must treat symptomatically while diagnostic clarity emerges over time.

Use provisional diagnoses when appropriate. "Rule out ADHD" or "Anxiety disorder, unspecified" acknowledge uncertainty while allowing treatment initiation. Revise diagnoses as information accumulates.

Comorbidity complicates everything. The child with autism, ADHD, anxiety, and intellectual disability needs integrated treatment considering all conditions. Prioritize by impairment but address interaction effects. ADHD medication might worsen anxiety. Anxiety treatment might improve attention.

Resource limitations affect treatment planning. The evidence-based treatment might be unavailable or unaffordable. Insurance might not cover recommended intensity. Families might lack transportation for multiple weekly sessions.

Be creative within constraints. Teletherapy expands access. Group treatment reduces costs. Training parents as co-therapists extends intervention into home. School-based services eliminate transportation barriers.

Family disagreement about diagnosis or treatment derails progress. Divorced parents might have opposing views. Cultural differences might create conflict about medication or therapy. Adolescents might refuse treatment parents want.

Address disagreements directly. Explore each person's concerns. Find common ground - everyone wants the child to suffer less. Sometimes agreeing on small steps forward works better than forcing comprehensive plans.

Practical Application

That thirteen-year-old from the opening? The comprehensive formulation revealed trauma-triggered ADHD symptoms exacerbated by learning disabilities within dysfunctional family system. Simply treating ADHD would have failed. Simply addressing trauma would have missed learning needs. Family therapy alone wouldn't address neurobiological factors.

The integrated treatment plan included trauma-focused CBT for PTSD, stimulant medication for ADHD, educational advocacy for learning accommodations, and structural family therapy for home chaos. SMART goals addressed each domain - reducing nightmares, improving homework completion, increasing reading level, and establishing consistent bedtime routine.

Three months later, progress was mixed. Trauma symptoms improved significantly. ADHD medication helped focus. School provided accommodations. But family chaos continued undermining progress. Treatment plan revision increased family therapy intensity and added parent coaching.

This iterative process - formulate, plan, implement, assess, revise - continues throughout treatment. No plan is perfect initially. Children change, families evolve, new information emerges. Flexible persistence, guided by thoughtful formulation and collaborative planning, leads to success.

Essential Principles for Success

Diagnostic formulation is more than listing problems - it's understanding how biological vulnerabilities, psychological processes, social contexts, and developmental factors interact to create this unique child's struggles. Take time to formulate thoroughly. Rush this step, and treatment fails.

Treatment planning must be truly collaborative. Children and families who help create plans follow them better. Even resistant adolescents engage more when their voice is heard. Imposed plans, however brilliant, usually fail.

SMART goals transform wishes into achievable targets. Vague goals lead to vague outcomes. Specific, measurable goals create accountability and demonstrate progress. Celebrate small victories building toward larger changes.

Match treatment to child, not child to treatment. The best evidence-based treatment delivered inflexibly helps no one. Adapt interventions for developmental stage, cultural background, family capacity, and individual preferences.

Documentation isn't paperwork - it's communication. Clear treatment plans align team members, inform coverage decisions, and guide care across transitions. Write plans others can understand and implement.

Stay flexible. Initial formulations and plans are hypotheses to test, not rigid prescriptions. When treatment stalls, reformulate. When goals are met, create new ones. When families struggle, adjust expectations. Persistence plus flexibility equals progress.

The science of diagnosis and the art of treatment planning merge in pediatric psychiatric nursing. Master both, and you'll transform complex presentations into understandable formulations and effective interventions. That's how confused, struggling children become clear diagnostic pictures with hopeful treatment paths.

Chapter 7: Psychotherapeutic Interventions Across Development

A four-year-old builds towers with blocks, then gleefully knocks them down. "That's what happens at my house," she says quietly. In another room, a ten-year-old practices deep breathing while holding an ice cube, learning to tolerate discomfort without panicking. Down the hall, a sixteen-year-old fills out a diary card tracking emotions, urges, and skills used. Three different ages, three different approaches, all working toward healing.

Psychotherapy with children and adolescents isn't just adult therapy made smaller. Each developmental stage requires distinct approaches, techniques, and adaptations. The intervention that works brilliantly for a teenager might be completely inappropriate for a preschooler. Understanding how to match therapeutic modalities to developmental capacity, presenting problems, and family context determines whether therapy becomes a transformative experience or another frustrating failure.

Early Childhood Interventions

Young children don't have the verbal skills or abstract thinking to engage in traditional talk therapy. They can't lie on a couch and free-associate about their mother. They can't identify cognitive distortions or challenge negative thoughts. But they can play, and through play, they reveal and heal their inner worlds.

Play therapy serves as the foundation for early childhood intervention. Children naturally use play to process experiences, express emotions, and practice new skills. In play therapy, toys become words and play becomes language. The child who can't verbalize abuse might reenact it with dolls. The one who can't express grief might bury toy animals repeatedly.

Non-directive play therapy lets the child lead. You provide a safe space with carefully selected toys - a dollhouse for family dynamics, puppets for storytelling, art supplies for expression, aggressive toys for anger release. The child chooses what to play, and you reflect their actions and feelings. "You're making the daddy doll hit the baby doll. The baby looks scared."

This reflection serves multiple purposes. It shows you're paying attention, validates the child's experience, and helps them develop emotional vocabulary. Over time, themes emerge. The child works through trauma, practices different outcomes, and develops mastery over overwhelming experiences.

Directive play therapy involves more therapist guidance. You might introduce specific activities targeting identified issues. The anxious child practices brave behavior with puppets. The aggressive child learns calming techniques through bubble-blowing. The grieving child creates memory books. You're still using play as the medium, but with therapeutic goals in mind.

Parent-Child Interaction Therapy (PCIT) revolutionized treatment for young children with behavioral problems. Instead of seeing the child alone, PCIT coaches parents in real-time through a bug-in-the-ear device while they interact with their child. It's like having a therapist whispering expert guidance during challenging parenting moments.

PCIT has two phases. Child-Directed Interaction (CDI) teaches parents to follow their child's lead in play, using specific skills acronymed PRIDE: Praise, Reflection, Imitation, Description, and Enthusiasm. Parents learn to ignore minor misbehavior while attending to positive behavior. "You're building a tall tower!" becomes more powerful than "Stop throwing blocks!"

Parent-Directed Interaction (PDI) adds effective limit-setting. Parents learn to give clear, age-appropriate commands and follow through consistently. They practice time-out procedures that actually work. The brilliance of PCIT lies in its specificity - parents know exactly what to say and do, removing guesswork from discipline.

Research shows PCIT reduces behavior problems more effectively than traditional therapy. But here's what's really happening - it's restructuring the parent-child relationship. Parents become more attuned, children feel more secure, and negative cycles break. The "bad" kid becomes a child whose needs are understood and met appropriately.

Behavioral interventions for young children focus on concrete, observable changes. Token economies use stickers or points to reinforce desired behaviors. Visual schedules help children anticipate transitions. Social stories teach appropriate behavior through simple narratives. These aren't bribes or manipulation - they're scaffolding for children whose brains haven't developed internal motivation and control.

The key with behavioral interventions is consistency and immediacy. Young children can't connect consequences to behaviors that happened hours ago. The reinforcement must come immediately - catch them being good and reward right away. The four-year-old who shares a toy gets a sticker immediately, not at the end of the day.

Environmental modifications often work better than trying to change the child directly. The hyperactive preschooler might need a sensory diet with regular movement breaks. The anxious child might need a quiet corner with calming materials. Sometimes changing the environment eliminates the need for behavioral intervention.

School-Age Interventions

School-age children can engage in more structured therapy, though modifications for concrete thinking remain necessary. They can identify feelings, understand cause-and-effect, and practice new skills, but abstract concepts still challenge them.

CBT adaptations for children make cognitive work concrete and engaging. Instead of thought logs, use thought bubbles drawn around cartoon characters. Replace abstract restructuring with "detective thinking" - gathering evidence for and against worried thoughts. The child afraid of dogs becomes a "dog detective," observing real dog behavior versus scary thoughts.

Behavioral experiments work particularly well with school-age children. The child who thinks everyone will laugh if they make mistakes tests this hypothesis in small ways. Start with low-risk situations - making a silly face with family - before progressing to classroom participation. Each experiment provides concrete evidence challenging anxious predictions.

Problem-solving skills training breaks down overwhelming situations into manageable steps. The child learns to identify problems, brainstorm solutions, evaluate options, try one, and assess results. This becomes a life skill extending beyond therapy. The child who learns problem-solving for friendship conflicts applies it to academic challenges.

Social skills training addresses the peer relationship difficulties common in school-age children. Many children with mental health issues struggle socially - anxiety makes them withdrawn, ADHD makes them impulsive, depression makes them irritable. Poor peer relationships then worsen mental health, creating vicious cycles.

Group-based social skills training allows real-time practice. Children learn to read social cues, join groups, handle disagreements, and maintain friendships. Role-playing provides safe practice before real-world application. The child who practices asking to join a game in therapy feels more confident on the playground.

But social skills aren't just behaviors to memorize. Context matters enormously. The joke that's funny with friends might be inappropriate in class. The assertiveness needed with bullies differs from negotiating with friends. Teaching social flexibility often matters more than specific skills.

Group therapy offers unique benefits for school-age children. Universality - discovering others share similar struggles - reduces shame and isolation. The anxious child learns they're not the only one who worries. The angry child sees others struggling with temper too.

Groups provide natural opportunities for peer feedback. Children often accept input from peers better than adults. When another child says, "That's annoying when you interrupt," it carries more weight than adult correction. Peers also model coping strategies more convincingly than adult demonstration.

Structured groups work best for this age. Clear rules, predictable activities, and consistent schedules help children feel safe. Unstructured process groups that work for adolescents overwhelm school-age children. They need activities, games, and concrete discussion topics.

Adolescent Interventions

Adolescents can engage in sophisticated therapy resembling adult treatment, but developmental considerations remain crucial. Identity formation, peer influence, and autonomy needs shape therapeutic approach.

CBT for adolescents addresses the abstract thinking and rumination characteristic of teenage depression and anxiety. Teenagers can identify thinking patterns, understand how thoughts influence feelings and behaviors, and actively challenge distortions. The depressed teen learns to recognize all-or-nothing thinking: "If I'm not perfect, I'm worthless."

But CBT with adolescents requires engagement strategies. Worksheets feel like homework. Instead, use technology - mood tracking apps, text message reminders, online thought logs. Make examples relevant - social media comparisons, academic pressure, relationship drama. The more therapy connects to their actual lives, the more they engage.

Behavioral activation particularly helps depressed adolescents who've withdrawn from everything. Start small - one pleasant activity daily - and build gradually. The teen who hasn't left their room in weeks won't suddenly become social butterflies. First goal: shower daily. Next: eat one meal with family. Gradually: text a friend.

Dialectical Behavior Therapy for Adolescents (DBT-A) adapts Linehan's model for teenagers struggling with emotion dysregulation, self-harm, and suicidality. The core principle - dialectics - resonates with adolescents navigating identity questions. They can be angry at parents AND love them. They can want independence AND need support.

DBT-A teaches four skill modules. Mindfulness helps teens observe emotions without being controlled by them. Distress tolerance provides alternatives to self-harm for managing overwhelming feelings. Emotion regulation helps understand and manage feeling states. Interpersonal effectiveness teaches asking for what they need while maintaining relationships.

The skills training group component of DBT-A provides peer support while learning. Teenagers practice skills together, share successes and failures, and normalize the struggle of managing intense emotions. Diary cards track skill use between sessions, creating accountability and self-awareness.

Individual therapy in DBT-A balances validation with change. "It makes complete sense you're angry about your parents' divorce. That really sucks. AND cutting yourself creates more problems. How can we help you express anger without hurting yourself?" This both/and approach respects their experience while promoting healthier coping.

Interpersonal Therapy for Adolescents (IPT-A) focuses on relationship problems contributing to depression. Adolescent depression often connects to interpersonal issues - grief, role disputes, role transitions, or interpersonal deficits. IPT-A addresses these directly rather than exploring childhood or changing thinking patterns.

The grieving teen works through loss - not just death but losses like parental divorce, friendship endings, or health changes. The teen in role dispute with parents negotiates independence versus family expectations. Role transitions might include starting high school, puberty, or family changes. Interpersonal deficits involve difficulty forming or maintaining relationships.

IPT-A is time-limited and focused, typically 12-16 sessions. This appeals to adolescents who want to see progress quickly. The structure provides containment for overwhelming feelings while the interpersonal focus addresses their primary developmental task - relationships.

Motivational interviewing works particularly well with ambivalent adolescents. Many teenagers don't want therapy, don't see problems, or feel forced by parents. Traditional confrontation triggers oppositional responses. Motivational interviewing rolls with resistance rather than opposing it.

"You don't think smoking weed is a problem. Tell me what you like about it." This unexpected response opens dialogue rather than shutting it down. Exploring ambivalence - "What's good about weed? What's not so good?" - helps teens recognize their own concerns without feeling lectured.

The key is genuine curiosity rather than hidden agenda. If teens sense you're manipulating them toward predetermined conclusions, they'll shut down. But when you're genuinely interested in their perspective, they often talk themselves into change. "I guess getting suspended did mess things up..."

Specialized Modalities

Some interventions work across developmental stages with appropriate modifications. These specialized approaches address specific issues like trauma, family dysfunction, or treatment-resistant conditions.

Trauma-Focused CBT (TF-CBT) helps children and adolescents process traumatic experiences. The components spell PRACTICE: Psychoeducation, Relaxation, Affective expression, Cognitive coping, Trauma narrative, In vivo mastery, Conjoint sessions, and Enhancing safety.

The trauma narrative component requires careful pacing. Children gradually approach trauma memories through drawing, writing, or talking. Starting with less distressing aspects, they slowly approach the worst moments. This graduated exposure, combined with cognitive processing, reduces trauma's power.

Parent involvement in TF-CBT is crucial. Parents learn about trauma's impact, manage their own distress, and support their child's healing. Conjoint sessions allow children to share their narrative with parents, often revealing previously unknown details. This shared understanding promotes family healing.

TF-CBT adapts to developmental level. Young children might use dolls to show what happened. School-age children might draw comic strips depicting their trauma and recovery. Adolescents might write songs or poetry. The narrative technique matters less than the processing it enables.

EMDR (Eye Movement Desensitization and Reprocessing) uses bilateral stimulation to process traumatic memories. While controversial, research supports its effectiveness with children and adolescents. The bilateral stimulation - originally eye movements, now often tapping or sounds - seems to facilitate trauma processing.

With children, EMDR requires creative adaptations. Instead of eye movements, they might drum alternately with both hands. Puppets on each hand can tell different parts of the story. The "butterfly hug" - crossing arms and alternately tapping shoulders - provides self-administered bilateral stimulation.

The key is making it developmentally appropriate and engaging. Young children need more preparation and shorter sessions. Adolescents might use technology - alternating tones through headphones while processing. The bilateral stimulation remains constant, but delivery adapts to development.

Family therapy recognizes that children's problems often reflect family system issues. The anxious child might be responding to parental conflict. The oppositional adolescent might be distracting from marital problems. Individual therapy without addressing family dynamics often fails.

Structural family therapy examines and adjusts family organization. Are boundaries appropriate? Is hierarchy clear? The child who's parentified - taking adult responsibilities - needs boundaries restored. Parents who've abdicated authority need empowerment to resume appropriate roles.

Strategic family therapy uses specific interventions to interrupt problematic patterns. Paradoxical interventions prescribe the symptom: "This week, have your temper tantrum every day at 4 PM for exactly 10 minutes." This transforms involuntary symptoms into choices, often eliminating them.

Narrative family therapy helps families rewrite their stories. Instead of being "the family with the problem child," they become "the family overcoming challenges together." This shift from problem-saturated to strength-based narratives transforms family identity and interactions.

Session Structure Across Development

Session structure varies dramatically by age, even with the same intervention. Understanding these structural needs ensures therapeutic engagement and effectiveness.

Early childhood sessions (45 minutes typical) might include:

- 5 minutes: Parent check-in without child
- 5 minutes: Transition and greeting with child
- 30 minutes: Play therapy or intervention
- 5 minutes: Clean-up and closure with child
- 5 minutes: Parent feedback and planning

The physical space matters enormously. Child-sized furniture, accessible toys, and clear boundaries create safety. Consistent session structure provides predictability anxious children need. The same opening song, closing ritual, or special goodbye creates containing rhythms.

School-age sessions (50 minutes typical) might include:

- 5 minutes: Check-in and agenda setting
- 10 minutes: Homework review or skill practice
- 25 minutes: Core therapeutic work
- 10 minutes: Planning and practice for coming week

School-age children benefit from visual aids tracking progress. Feeling thermometers, worry scales, or behavior charts make abstract progress concrete. Session notebooks where children record insights and homework maintain continuity between sessions.

Adolescent sessions (50-60 minutes typical) need flexibility:

- 10 minutes: Check-in and urgent issues
- 30 minutes: Therapeutic work
- 10 minutes: Skill practice or planning

Adolescents might need entire sessions processing crises. The teen who just broke up with their first love can't focus on homework review. Flexibility while maintaining structure respects developmental needs while ensuring progress.

Activity Guides and Engagement

Engaging activities make therapy effective and even enjoyable. Generic worksheets rarely engage. Creative, developmentally matched activities maintain therapeutic engagement.

For young children:

- Feelings faces plates: Paper plates decorated as emotions
- Worry dolls: Tiny dolls that "hold" worries at night
- Calm-down bottles: Glitter bottles for self-soothing
- Bravery badges: Earned for facing fears
- Anger volcano: Showing anger building and erupting

For school-age children:

- Worry warriors: Characters fighting anxiety monsters
- Thought detective worksheets: Investigating worried thoughts
- Coping cards: Decorated index cards with personal strategies
- Feelings journal: Daily emotion tracking with colors/stickers
- Problem-solving wheels: Spinning options for solutions

For adolescents:

- Playlist therapy: Songs representing different emotions
- Meme-making: Creating memes about their experiences
- Vision boards: Future goals and identity exploration
- Slam poetry: Writing and performing about struggles
- Photography projects: Capturing emotions through images

Fidelity and Adaptation Balance

Treatment fidelity - delivering interventions as designed - matters for effectiveness. But rigid manualization ignores individual differences. The art lies in maintaining core components while adapting delivery.

Core components are non-negotiable. TF-CBT requires trauma narrative work. DBT requires all four skill modules. PCIT requires both CDI and PDI phases. Skipping core components means you're not delivering the actual treatment.

But delivery can adapt. The trauma narrative might be spoken, written, drawn, or acted out. DBT skills might be taught through games, apps, or traditional worksheets. PCIT might happen in clinic, home, or via telehealth. Flexibility in delivery maintains engagement while preserving effectiveness.

Cultural adaptations enhance rather than compromise fidelity. Using culturally relevant examples, incorporating family values, and respecting communication styles improves engagement. The Latino family might need *familismo* incorporated. The Asian family might prefer indirect communication about emotions.

Documentation ensures both fidelity and adaptation tracking. Note which components were delivered and how they were adapted. "Completed trauma narrative through sand tray rather than verbal processing due to selective mutism" maintains accountability while honoring individual needs.

Real-World Implementation Challenges

Theory meets reality when implementing interventions. The perfect protocol encounters imperfect situations requiring clinical judgment and creativity.

Engagement challenges are common. The child who won't talk, the teenager who attends but won't participate, the family that misses half their appointments. Before labeling as "resistant," explore barriers. Transportation? Scheduling? Cultural mismatch? Addressing practical barriers often resolves "resistance."

Sometimes the intervention-problem mismatch causes disengagement. CBT won't help if the real issue is family chaos. Individual therapy won't work if the system maintains symptoms. Recognizing when to switch approaches requires humility and flexibility.

Comorbidity complicates intervention selection. The child with ADHD, anxiety, and trauma needs integrated treatment. Starting with one condition while ignoring others often fails. Sometimes you need to address everything simultaneously; sometimes sequencing makes sense.

Resource limitations affect real-world delivery. The evidence-based treatment might require two therapists, specialized training, or materials your setting lacks. Creative adaptations maintain quality within constraints. Group delivery reduces costs. Peer providers extend reach. Technology enables access.

Crisis interruptions disrupt protocol adherence. The session planned for cognitive restructuring becomes suicide assessment. The family session becomes CPS reporting. Maintaining therapeutic progress while managing crises requires flexibility and persistence.

Essential Practice Principles

Developmental attunement matters more than perfect protocol adherence. The intervention that's evidence-based for an age group might not fit this specific child. The mature ten-year-old might benefit from adolescent approaches. The delayed teenager might need child-oriented interventions.

Relationship remains the foundation. The best intervention delivered without genuine connection fails. Children and adolescents have excellent authenticity detectors. They know when you're going through motions versus genuinely caring. Prioritize relationship even when it means deviating from protocol.

Family involvement usually improves outcomes, but involvement looks different across development and situations. The preschooler needs parents as co-therapists. The adolescent needs privacy with appropriate parent inclusion. The foster child might need careful navigation of multiple "families."

Cultural humility enhances every intervention. Your evidence-based treatment was likely developed on specific populations. Assuming universal application ignores cultural variation in emotional expression, help-seeking, and healing. Stay curious about how culture influences this specific child's experience and needs.

Progress isn't always linear. The child making steady progress suddenly regresses. The adolescent who seemed stable suddenly crises. Development itself creates instability - new cognitive abilities enable new worries, hormonal changes destabilize mood. Expect zigzags rather than straight lines.

The intervention is just one part of healing. Therapy provides tools, insights, and support, but real change happens between sessions. How parents respond to meltdowns, how teachers handle anxiety, how peers include or exclude - these daily interactions often matter more than weekly therapy.

Your role shifts across development and intervention. Sometimes you're teacher providing psychoeducation. Sometimes you're coach building skills. Sometimes you're witness to pain. Sometimes you're cheerleader celebrating progress. Flexibility in role while maintaining boundaries enables therapeutic effectiveness.

The best intervention is one the child and family will actually use. The theoretically superior treatment that feels wrong to them won't help. The "good enough" intervention they embrace works better than perfect protocols they resist. Match intervention to family, not family to intervention.

Chapter 8: Psychopharmacology in Pediatric Populations

The mother sits across from you, tears streaming down her face. Her eight-year-old son has tried three different therapists, two social skills groups, and a special behavior plan at school. Nothing has helped his severe ADHD. He can't make friends, can't learn, can't even play soccer because he can't follow the game. "I swore I'd never medicate my child," she says, "but watching him suffer is killing me. Will medication change who he is? Will it stunt his growth? Am I being a bad parent?"

These agonizing decisions face families every day. Psychiatric medications for children remain controversial, feared, misunderstood, and sometimes desperately needed. As a pediatric psychiatric nurse, you'll guide families through these decisions, monitor medication effects, manage side effects, and help distinguish between reasonable caution and harmful medication stigma. This requires understanding not just what medications do, but how developing bodies and brains respond differently than adults.

Pediatric Pharmacology Principles

"Start low, go slow" becomes your mantra in pediatric psychopharmacology. Children aren't small adults - their bodies process medications differently, their brains respond uniquely, and their developmental stage influences everything from absorption to adverse effects.

Pharmacokinetics in children - how bodies process medications - varies dramatically by age. Infants have immature liver enzymes, affecting metabolism. Toddlers might metabolize certain drugs faster than adults, requiring more frequent dosing. Adolescents going through puberty experience hormonal influences on drug metabolism. Body composition matters too - children have higher water-to-fat ratios than adults, affecting drug distribution.

Absorption differs as well. Gastric pH changes throughout childhood, affecting oral medication absorption. Skin permeability in young children increases topical absorption. Even something as simple as crushing pills for children who can't swallow tablets can alter absorption rates.

The blood-brain barrier, more permeable in young children, allows greater CNS penetration of medications. This might mean more effectiveness but also more side effects. The developing brain shows plasticity that can enhance therapeutic effects but also vulnerability to adverse impacts.

Pharmacodynamics - how medications affect the body - also varies developmentally. Neurotransmitter systems develop at different rates. The dopamine system peaks in adolescence, possibly explaining why stimulants work differently in teenagers versus younger children. Serotonin receptors change throughout development, affecting antidepressant response.

Receptor sensitivity changes with age. Young children might be more sensitive to certain effects but less to others. The six-year-old might need tiny doses of medication that barely touch adult depression. The teenager might need doses approaching or exceeding adult ranges.

Starting low means beginning with the smallest possible effective dose. For some medications, this means quarter or half the typical starting dose. You can always increase, but you can't take back adverse effects from starting too high. That traumatic first experience with medication might create resistance to all future trials.

Going slow means gradual titration based on response and tolerability. Increase by small increments every week or two, not daily. Watch for both therapeutic effects and side effects. The child whose behavior improves but stops eating needs dose adjustment, not discontinuation.

Off-label prescribing is the norm, not exception, in pediatric psychiatry. Most psychiatric medications lack FDA approval for children, especially for specific age groups. This doesn't mean they're unsafe or ineffective - it means companies haven't conducted expensive pediatric trials.

But off-label use requires extra vigilance. You're relying on clinical experience, smaller studies, and extrapolation from adult data. Informed consent becomes crucial. Parents need to understand you're using clinical judgment, not FDA guidance. Document reasoning carefully.

The younger the child, the less evidence typically exists. Preschool psychopharmacology relies heavily on expert consensus and careful monitoring. That three-year-old with severe ADHD might benefit from stimulants, but you're in relatively uncharted territory.

Antidepressants and the Black Box Warning

The black box warning about increased suicidality in youth taking antidepressants terrifies parents and prescribers alike. But understanding what this actually means - and doesn't mean - helps guide rational decision-making.

The warning emerged from meta-analyses showing about 4% of youth on antidepressants experienced increased suicidal ideation versus 2% on placebo. That's a doubling of relative risk but still low absolute risk. No completed suicides occurred in these trials. The risk appears highest in the first few weeks, particularly if activation occurs before mood improvement.

But here's what often gets missed - untreated depression carries far higher suicide risk than antidepressants. The teenager with severe depression faces about 15% lifetime suicide risk without treatment.

Avoiding antidepressants due to black box fears might increase rather than decrease danger.

SSRIs (Selective Serotonin Reuptake Inhibitors) remain first-line for pediatric depression and anxiety. Fluoxetine has the most evidence and FDA approval for childhood depression. Its long half-life provides built-in taper if doses are missed. Sertraline and escitalopram also show good evidence, with FDA approval for OCD and depression respectively.

Starting doses should be half or less of adult doses. Fluoxetine might start at 5-10mg, not 20mg. Sertraline might begin at 12.5-25mg, not 50mg. This reduces activation risk - that uncomfortable energized feeling preceding mood improvement.

Activation is the most concerning short-term side effect. The child becomes agitated, impulsive, or hypomanic. They might feel "crawling out of their skin." This isn't true mania but rather a medication side effect requiring dose reduction or discontinuation. Parents need clear warnings about activation and instructions to call immediately if it occurs.

Other common side effects include GI upset (usually transient), headaches, sleep changes, and sexual side effects in adolescents. Weight changes vary - some children lose appetite initially, others gain weight long-term. Growth should be monitored but isn't typically affected.

SNRIs (Serotonin-Norepinephrine Reuptake Inhibitors) like duloxetine might help when SSRIs fail. The norepinephrine component might improve energy and focus. But SNRIs can increase blood pressure and heart rate, requiring monitoring.

Atypical antidepressants each have unique profiles. Bupropion helps depression with ADHD or when avoiding weight gain matters. But it lowers seizure threshold and can increase anxiety. Mirtazapine helps depression with insomnia or poor appetite but causes sedation and weight gain.

98

ADHD Medications

ADHD medications transform lives when used appropriately. The child who couldn't sit still, couldn't make friends, couldn't learn suddenly can engage with their world. But these powerful medications require careful selection, titration, and monitoring.

Stimulants - methylphenidate and amphetamine preparations - remain first-line treatment with 70-80% response rates. They work by increasing dopamine and norepinephrine in prefrontal cortex, improving attention, impulse control, and executive function.

The methylphenidate family includes immediate-release (Ritalin), extended-release (Concerta), and various other formulations. Amphetamines include mixed amphetamine salts (Adderall) and lisdexamfetamine (Vyvanse). Despite chemical differences, effectiveness is similar - choice depends on duration needed and individual response.

Starting stimulants requires establishing baseline vital signs, height, weight, and appetite. Start with immediate-release formulations to assess response and tolerability before moving to longer-acting preparations. A typical starting dose might be 5mg methylphenidate twice daily or 2.5-5mg amphetamine once daily.

Titration occurs weekly, increasing by small increments until optimal response without significant side effects. The "right" dose varies enormously - some children need tiny doses, others need maximum FDA-approved amounts. Body weight doesn't predict dose needs.

Common side effects include appetite suppression, sleep difficulty, and mood changes. Appetite typically returns partially with time. Giving medication after breakfast, providing high-calorie snacks, and "drug holidays" on weekends might help. Sleep improves with earlier dosing and good sleep hygiene.

The "zombie" effect parents fear - emotional blunting or personality change - suggests dose is too high or wrong medication. Children should be themselves, just more focused. If spark disappears, reduce dose or switch preparations.

Growth suppression averages about 1cm over childhood with continuous use. Most children catch up during drug holidays or after discontinuation. Monitor growth curves, but don't discontinue effective treatment for minimal height differences.

Non-stimulants provide alternatives when stimulants fail or cause intolerable side effects. Atomoxetine (Strattera) works through norepinephrine reuptake inhibition. It takes weeks to work versus hours for stimulants. Start at 0.5mg/kg daily, increasing gradually to 1.2mg/kg.

Atomoxetine doesn't cause appetite suppression or insomnia like stimulants. But it can cause nausea, fatigue, and rarely, liver problems or suicidal ideation. It's particularly useful when anxiety coexists with ADHD or when substance abuse risk concerns exist.

Alpha-2 agonists - guanfacine and clonidine - help hyperactivity and impulsivity more than inattention. They're particularly useful for aggression, tics, or sleep problems accompanying ADHD. Start with tiny doses (0.5mg guanfacine or 0.05mg clonidine) at bedtime, as sedation is common initially.

Antipsychotics and Metabolic Monitoring

Second-generation antipsychotics revolutionized treatment of childhood aggression, bipolar disorder, and psychosis. But their metabolic side effects create new problems requiring vigilant monitoring.

Indications keep expanding beyond psychosis. Risperidone and aripiprazole have FDA approval for irritability in autism. Multiple antipsychotics are approved for pediatric bipolar disorder. They're used off-label for severe aggression, DMDD, and treatment-resistant depression.

But antipsychotics aren't benign. Weight gain averages 5-10 pounds in the first months. Some children gain much more. Olanzapine and clozapine cause the most weight gain; aripiprazole and ziprasidone the least. But individual variation is huge.

Metabolic syndrome - obesity, diabetes, dyslipidemia, hypertension - can develop even in children. The eight-year-old started on risperidone for aggression might develop type 2 diabetes by adolescence. These aren't just cosmetic concerns but serious health risks.

Baseline metabolic monitoring must occur before starting antipsychotics: weight, height, BMI, waist circumference, blood pressure, fasting glucose, and lipid panel. Family history of diabetes or cardiovascular disease increases risk.

Ongoing monitoring continues regularly - monthly weights for three months, then quarterly. Metabolic panels every three months initially, then every six months. Any rapid weight gain or metabolic changes require intervention.

But monitoring without intervention is meaningless. If a child gains 10 pounds in two months, you can't just document it. Consider dose reduction, medication switch, or adding metformin. Refer to nutrition and exercise programs. Address it aggressively before metabolic syndrome establishes.

Movement disorders represent another concern. Acute dystonia - sudden muscle spasms - terrifies children and families. Educate about this rare but dramatic side effect. Benztropine or diphenhydramine provides rapid relief.

Tardive dyskinesia - involuntary movements after prolonged use - might be permanent. Regular AIMS (Abnormal Involuntary

Movement Scale) assessments detect early signs. The earlier caught, the more likely reversibility with discontinuation.

Hyperprolactinemia from dopamine blockade causes various problems. Galactorrhea embarrasses adolescents. Amenorrhea concerns parents. Gynecomastia devastates teenage boys. Check prolactin levels if symptoms occur. Switching to aripiprazole or adding low-dose aripiprazole might help.

Mood Stabilizers

Mood stabilizers treat pediatric bipolar disorder, severe mood dysregulation, and sometimes aggression. But they require extensive monitoring and carry significant risks.

Lithium, the oldest mood stabilizer, remains effective for classic bipolar disorder. But pediatric use requires careful consideration. Therapeutic windows are narrow - too little doesn't work, too much becomes toxic.

Start lithium at 300mg daily or 10mg/kg, divided into two or three doses. Increase gradually every 5-7 days based on levels and response. Therapeutic levels (0.8-1.2 mEq/L) must be monitored regularly - weekly initially, then monthly when stable.

Side effects at therapeutic levels include tremor, increased thirst/urination, weight gain, and cognitive dulling. The straight-A student who becomes C-student on lithium faces difficult decisions. Sometimes lower levels (0.6-0.8) provide benefit with fewer side effects.

Toxicity is the major concern. Dehydration from sports, vomiting from stomach flu, or drug interactions can push levels dangerous. Symptoms include severe tremor, confusion, and seizures. Families need detailed education about maintaining hydration and recognizing toxicity.

Long-term concerns include thyroid and kidney effects. Monitor TSH and creatinine regularly. After years of use, some develop hypothyroidism or reduced kidney function. These aren't inevitable but require vigilance.

Anticonvulsant mood stabilizers provide alternatives to lithium. Valproic acid helps mania and mixed states but requires extensive monitoring. Baseline liver functions, CBC, and pregnancy testing (it causes severe birth defects) are essential.

Weight gain with valproate can be severe. PCOS (polycystic ovary syndrome) develops in some females. Hair loss distresses teenagers. Tremor and cognitive effects occur. Despite FDA approval for adult bipolar disorder, pediatric evidence is limited.

Lamotrigine helps bipolar depression more than mania. But Stevens-Johnson syndrome - a potentially fatal rash - requires extremely slow titration. Start at 25mg every other day, increasing by 25mg weekly. Any rash requires immediate evaluation.

Carbamazepine, once commonly used, has fallen from favor due to drug interactions and monitoring requirements. Oxcarbazepine has fewer interactions but limited evidence. Both can cause hyponatremia and require regular monitoring.

Special Considerations

Certain situations require extra caution and modified approaches in pediatric psychopharmacology.

Pregnancy in adolescents creates agonizing dilemmas. Most psychotropics carry some fetal risk, but untreated mental illness also threatens mother and baby. The severely depressed pregnant teenager needs treatment, but what's safest?

SSRIs, especially sertraline, have extensive pregnancy data showing relative safety. Small risks of cardiac defects, persistent pulmonary hypertension, and neonatal withdrawal exist but are rare. Untreated depression carries risks of poor prenatal care, substance use, and suicide.

Mood stabilizers pose bigger challenges. Lithium causes cardiac defects (though less than previously thought). Valproate causes neural tube defects and developmental delays. Lamotrigine appears safer but isn't risk-free. Sometimes switching to antipsychotics during pregnancy makes sense.

The key is shared decision-making. Present risks honestly - both of treatment and non-treatment. Document discussions thoroughly. Coordinate with obstetrics. Plan for postpartum - a high-risk period for psychiatric decompensation.

Substance use commonly co-occurs with psychiatric disorders in adolescents. Stimulants might be diverted or abused. Benzodiazepines risk dependence. Even antidepressants can be misused. But undertreating ADHD or anxiety might drive self-medication with dangerous substances.

Long-acting or abuse-deterrent formulations help. Vyvanse requires enzymatic conversion, preventing snorting or injecting. Atomoxetine lacks abuse potential. Drug testing might be appropriate but can damage therapeutic relationships if handled punitively.

Address substance use directly rather than hoping medications fix everything. Integrated treatment for co-occurring disorders works better than sequential treatment. The teenager using marijuana for anxiety needs both anxiety treatment and substance counseling.

Discontinuation requires as much care as initiation. Abrupt cessation causes withdrawal symptoms easily mistaken for relapse. SSRIs (except fluoxetine) cause discontinuation syndrome - flu-like symptoms, brain zaps, mood changes. Taper gradually over weeks to months.

The question of when to discontinue challenges everyone. After 6-12 months of stability? Never if it's working? During summer break? There's no universal answer. Consider severity of original symptoms, number of episodes, side effects, and family preference.

Some children need medication briefly during crisis. Others need long-term treatment for chronic conditions. The child who needed stimulants in elementary school might not in high school. The teenager with recurrent depression might need lifelong treatment. Regular reassessment, not assumptions, should guide decisions.

Practical Medication Management

Real-world medication management goes beyond prescribing. It involves education, monitoring, advocacy, and support through the entire medication journey.

Initial education sets the foundation. Use simple language: "This medicine helps your brain make more happy chemicals." Address specific fears: "No, this won't change your personality." Provide written information at appropriate reading levels.

Involve children appropriately in discussions. The six-year-old needs to know they're taking medicine to help them pay attention. The sixteen-year-old should understand risks, benefits, and alternatives. Respect developing autonomy while maintaining safety.

Adherence challenges are normal, not defiant. Pills taste bad. Side effects are unpleasant. Teenagers forget or rebel. Parents disagree about medication. Instead of lecturing about non-compliance, explore barriers collaboratively.

Practical solutions help: pill organizers, phone reminders, pairing with routine activities (brushing teeth), long-acting formulations to avoid school doses. Sometimes changing preparation helps - liquid, chewable, or patch instead of pills.

Monitoring extends beyond side effects. Track target symptoms systematically. Use rating scales - Vanderbilt for ADHD, PHQ-9A for depression. Graph changes over time. This objective data guides decisions better than vague impressions.

But don't just monitor problems. Track improvements too. Celebrate the first good report card on stimulants. Note the return of laughter on antidepressants. Document the decrease in meltdowns on mood stabilizers. Progress motivates continuation through difficult side effects.

Collaboration with other providers ensures comprehensive care. The prescriber needs to know about therapy progress. The therapist needs to understand medication effects. The school needs appropriate information to support the child. The pediatrician monitors growth and health impacts.

But maintain appropriate boundaries. The school doesn't need to know diagnoses or medications unless parents consent. Focus on functional needs: "This student needs movement breaks" rather than "This student takes ADHD medication."

Looking Forward

That mother from the opening? After careful discussion, her son started low-dose methylphenidate. The first week brought mild appetite suppression but dramatic improvement in focus. By week three, he completed homework independently for the first time. After two months, he was invited to a birthday party - his first ever.

His growth slowed slightly, but his confidence soared. Medication didn't change who he was - it revealed who he'd always been underneath the ADHD chaos. Combined with behavioral therapy and school support, medication enabled him to succeed academically, socially, and emotionally.

Not every medication story ends so positively. Some children don't respond. Others experience intolerable side effects. Finding the right medication at the right dose takes patience, persistence, and sometimes multiple trials. But when it works, psychiatric medication can be literally life-saving.

Your role as a pediatric psychiatric nurse involves more than managing medications. You're educator, advocate, monitor, and support. You help families navigate the complex decision to medicate. You distinguish between reasonable caution and harmful stigma. You monitor for both benefits and risks. You celebrate improvements and problem-solve challenges.

Most importantly, you recognize that medication is just one tool in comprehensive treatment. Pills don't teach skills, resolve trauma, or fix family dysfunction. But they might provide the stability needed to engage in therapy, succeed in school, and develop relationships. Used thoughtfully as part of integrated treatment, psychopharmacology helps children and adolescents reach their full potential.

Chapter 9: Crisis Intervention and Safety Management

The call comes at 2 AM. A fifteen-year-old on your unit is in the quiet room, screaming and throwing herself against the walls. She'd been doing well until another patient mentioned suicide at dinner, triggering memories of finding her father's body last year. The night staff look to you - the charge nurse - for guidance. Do you call for restraints? Administer PRN medication? Call security? Or is there another way?

Crisis moments like these test everything you know about pediatric psychiatric nursing. In seconds, you must assess danger, choose interventions, and act decisively while maintaining therapeutic relationships. The wrong response escalates situations, traumatizes children, and destroys trust. The right response de-escalates danger, preserves dignity, and can even become therapeutic breakthrough.

De-escalation by Developmental Stage

De-escalation isn't a single technique but a collection of approaches tailored to developmental capacity, individual needs, and specific situations. What calms a five-year-old might infuriate a fifteen-year-old. Understanding developmental differences in crisis response guides effective intervention.

Early childhood de-escalation requires understanding that young children can't regulate emotions independently. Their prefrontal cortex - the brain's control center - literally hasn't developed enough. When a preschooler melts down, they're not choosing defiance; they're drowning in feelings too big for their small bodies.

Physical proximity matters enormously with young children, but approach carefully. Quick movements or looming over them triggers

108

fight-or-flight responses. Instead, get on their level - kneel or sit. Keep your body relaxed and open. Your calm nervous system helps regulate theirs through co-regulation.

Use simple, concrete language. "You're mad the blocks fell down" works better than "Let's discuss your frustration." Reflect their emotions simply: "Mad, mad, MAD!" This shows you understand without adding verbal complexity they can't process when distressed.

Sensory interventions work well for young children. Offer a weighted blanket, play calming music, dim lights, or provide fidgets. Some children need movement - jumping on a trampoline or pushing against walls. Others need containment - a quiet corner with soft pillows.

Distraction isn't cheating; it's developmentally appropriate. The four-year-old screaming about leaving might calm when you notice their sparkly shoes. "Wow, do those shoes make you run super fast?" This isn't dismissing their feelings but helping their limited attention shift from distress.

School-age de-escalation acknowledges growing autonomy while recognizing continued need for adult support. These children have more emotional vocabulary and some self-regulation skills, but they still need scaffolding during crises.

Give choices within limits. "You can take space in the quiet room or walk with me" provides control without abandoning structure. Avoid ultimatums unless absolutely necessary. "You need to stop NOW or else..." escalates rather than calms.

Use their developing logical thinking. "When you throw chairs, people get scared. What else could you do when you're this angry?" This engages their problem-solving rather than just imposing solutions.

Validate their experience while maintaining boundaries. "I understand you're furious about the level drop. Being angry makes sense. AND throwing things isn't safe." This both/and approach respects their feelings while addressing behavior.

Privacy becomes important. The school-age child mortified by public meltdown might calm faster in private. Move to a quiet space if possible. Lower your voice so others can't hear. Protect their dignity while maintaining safety.

Adolescent de-escalation respects their near-adult cognitive abilities while remembering their still-developing emotional regulation. Teenagers in crisis need to maintain face while accepting help - a delicate balance.

Approach with respect and authenticity. Teenagers detect condescension immediately. "I can see you're really struggling right now. What would be helpful?" beats "Now, now, let's calm down." Treat them as partners in de-escalation, not problems to manage.

Give space initially. The agitated teenager might need physical distance to avoid feeling trapped. Stand at an angle rather than face-to-face. Keep exits visible. Say something like, "I'm going to stay over here, but I'm here when you're ready to talk."

Acknowledge their autonomy. "You're in control of your choices here. I can't make you calm down. But I'm wondering if there's something that might help you feel less awful right now?" This paradoxically often leads to accepting help.

Use their abstract thinking abilities. "I notice this started after group therapy. Is this connected to what we discussed?" Help them make connections between triggers and responses. This builds insight alongside de-escalation.

Universal De-escalation Principles

Regardless of age, certain principles apply to all crisis de-escalation.

Your calm is contagious. If you're anxious, aggressive, or frustrated, the child will escalate. Take a breath before engaging. Check your own emotional state. If you can't be calm, tag someone else in. Your regulated nervous system is your most powerful de-escalation tool.

Lower the stimulation. Reduce noise, dim lights, clear crowds. The overwhelmed nervous system needs less input, not more. That means using fewer words, softer voice, slower movements. Sometimes silence is the best intervention.

Validate before redirecting. "You're really angry" must come before "Let's try deep breathing." If children don't feel heard, they'll escalate to make you understand. Validation doesn't mean agreeing - it means acknowledging their experience.

Maintain safety without punishment. Removing dangerous objects isn't consequence - it's safety. Moving to a quiet room isn't punishment - it's reducing stimulation. Frame interventions as help, not discipline: "I need to keep everyone safe, including you."

Know when to disengage. Sometimes your presence escalates rather than calms. The child who screams louder when you approach might need space. "I'm going to give you a few minutes. I'll check back soon." This isn't abandonment but strategic disengagement.

Suicide Prevention and Safety Planning

Suicide is the second leading cause of death in youth aged 10-24. Every crisis assessment must include suicide screening, even when it seems unlikely. The quiet, compliant child might be at highest risk.

The ASQ (Ask Suicide-Screening Questions) provides validated screening for youth 8 and older:

1. In the past few weeks, have you wished you were dead?

2. In the past few weeks, have you felt that you or your family would be better off if you were dead?
3. In the past week, have you been having thoughts about killing yourself?
4. Have you ever tried to kill yourself?
5. Are you having thoughts of killing yourself right now?

Any "yes" requires further assessment. Don't panic, but don't minimize. The child who says "sometimes I wish I wouldn't wake up" needs as much attention as one with a specific plan.

The BSSA (Brief Suicide Safety Assessment) follows positive screens, assessing:

- Frequency and duration of suicidal thoughts
- Suicide plan and intent
- Access to means
- Past attempts and their lethality
- Protective factors and reasons for living

A child with passive death wishes, no plan, and strong protective factors might be safe for outpatient treatment. One with specific plan, intent, and means needs immediate hospitalization. Most fall somewhere between, requiring clinical judgment.

Safety planning collaborates with youth to create concrete strategies for managing suicidal crises. Unlike no-suicide contracts (which don't work), safety plans provide actual tools.

Warning signs come first. "What tells you the thoughts are starting?" Maybe it's isolation urges, specific thoughts, or physical sensations. The teenager who recognizes early warnings can intervene before crisis peaks.

Internal coping strategies follow. "What can you do alone to feel better?" This might be music, drawing, exercise, or specific apps. These strategies won't solve everything but might prevent escalation.

Social contacts for distraction come next. "Who can you talk to without discussing problems?" Sometimes just human connection without heavy processing helps. Friends who make them laugh, family members who provide normalcy.

Social contacts for help include people they can discuss suicidal thoughts with. This might be different from distraction contacts. The friend who's fun might not handle crisis disclosure well.

Professional contacts include therapist, psychiatrist, and crisis hotline numbers. Make these concrete: program numbers into their phone, write them on cards, ensure they're accessible during crisis when thinking becomes difficult.

Environmental safety involves removing or securing means. Lock up medications, remove firearms, restrict access to sharps. This isn't foolproof but adds barriers during impulsive moments. Most youth suicide attempts are impulsive with less than 10 minutes planning.

The Safety Plan Intervention (SPI) structures this process:

Step 1: Warning signs

- "When I start thinking everyone would be better off without me"
- "When I can't get out of bed for two days"
- "When I start giving things away"

Step 2: Internal coping strategies

- "Listen to my calm-down playlist"
- "Use my DBT skills"
- "Go for a run"

Step 3: People and places for distraction

- "Text Josh about video games"
- "Go to the library"

- "Call grandma"

Step 4: People to ask for help

- "Mom - even if it's the middle of the night"
- "Mrs. Johnson, school counselor"
- "Best friend Sarah"

Step 5: Professionals to contact

- Therapist (include actual number)
- Crisis hotline: 988
- Emergency department

Step 6: Making environment safe

- "Give mom my pills to lock up"
- "Stay out of the garage where dad's tools are"
- "Have someone else hold my razor"

Managing Aggressive Behavior Without Restraints

Physical restraints traumatize children, injure staff, and often escalate rather than resolve situations. The goal is preventing aggression, and when it occurs, managing it with minimal restrictiveness.

Environmental prevention reduces aggression triggers. Crowded spaces, loud noises, unclear expectations, and unpredictable schedules trigger fight-or-flight responses. Create calm environments with clear structure, predictable routines, and spaces for retreat.

Observe patterns. Does aggression happen during transitions? Before visits? After phone calls? Identifying patterns enables proactive intervention. The child who always escalates after family therapy might need extra support scheduled immediately after.

Early intervention catches escalation before violence. Watch for warning signs - clenched fists, pacing, raised voice, facial flushing. Intervene at first signs rather than waiting for full escalation.

Offer choices and control. "I can see you're getting upset. Would you like to take space or talk about it?" This respects autonomy while providing support. The child who feels trapped becomes dangerous; one with options often chooses well.

Use distraction and redirection. "Before we deal with that, can you help me with something?" Sometimes breaking the escalation cycle prevents aggression. This isn't avoiding issues but strategic timing.

When aggression occurs, safety comes first. Clear the area of others and dangerous objects. Don't crowd the aggressive child - this escalates panic. Create space while maintaining visual contact.

Use calm, simple directives. "Put down the chair" works better than lengthy explanations. Avoid arguing or reasoning during acute aggression - the thinking brain is offline. Just focus on immediate safety.

Team response should be coordinated, not chaotic. Designate one person as lead communicator. Others maintain safety perimeter. Too many people talking creates confusion and escalation.

Physical intervention as last resort follows specific protocols. Use the least restrictive method possible. Physical escort (walking with child) before physical restraint. Brief holds before extended restraints. Always reassess whether less restriction would work.

If restraint becomes necessary, use trained techniques minimizing injury risk. Never put pressure on chest, neck, or back. Monitor breathing constantly. Release as soon as safely possible. Document thoroughly including attempts at less restrictive interventions.

Debrief after every restraint. What triggered escalation? What interventions were tried? What worked or didn't? How did the child experience it? Without learning from each incident, patterns repeat.

Collaborative Crisis Management

Crisis management extends beyond your facility. Effective response requires coordination with schools, emergency services, families, and community providers.

School collaboration prevents and manages crises. Share crisis plans with appropriate school personnel (with consent). The school needs to know warning signs, effective interventions, and when to call for help.

Create re-entry plans after crisis hospitalizations. The child returning after suicide attempt needs supported transition. Maybe shortened days initially, check-ins with counselor, modified academics. Throwing them back into the same environment that triggered crisis invites relapse.

Train school personnel in de-escalation. Teachers who understand trauma responses, emotional dysregulation, and basic de-escalation prevent unnecessary emergency calls. A five-minute meltdown doesn't require police if staff know how to respond.

Emergency service coordination ensures appropriate response. Develop relationships with local emergency departments and mobile crisis teams. They need to understand your population and capabilities.

Create transfer protocols. When you send a child to emergency, what information goes with them? Medication list, crisis plan, contact numbers, recent events. Emergency departments overwhelmed with limited psychiatric knowledge need your expertise.

Train emergency responders about pediatric psychiatric crises. Police responding to psychiatric emergencies need understanding that these are ill children, not criminals. Advocate for Crisis Intervention Team (CIT) training in your community.

Family involvement during crisis requires balance. Families provide crucial information and support but might also trigger escalation. Assess each situation individually.

Some children calm immediately with parent presence. Others escalate dramatically. Know patterns for each child. The teenager who becomes violent when mom visits might need careful planning for family involvement during crisis.

Coach families in crisis response. Teach them de-escalation techniques, safety planning, and when to seek help. The family that knows how to respond prevents emergencies. But also validate when they need professional help - not every crisis should be managed at home.

Crisis Prevention Through Trauma-Informed Care

Many crises stem from trauma responses. Understanding behavior through a trauma lens transforms crisis intervention from managing problems to healing wounds.

Recognize trauma triggers. The child who escalates during shift change might be triggered by abandonment fears. The teenager who becomes aggressive when touched might be reliving abuse. Behavioral crises often represent trauma reenactment.

Create trauma-informed environments. Predictable routines reduce anxiety. Clear communication prevents surprises. Choice and control counter helplessness. These environmental modifications prevent many crises.

Teach regulation skills proactively. Don't wait for crisis to teach coping. Regular practice when calm builds skills for difficult

117

moments. The child who practices deep breathing daily can access it during distress.

Sensory modulation prevents escalation. Weighted blankets, fidgets, music, movement - these tools help children regulate before crisis. Create sensory kits individualized to each child's preferences.

Build distress tolerance. Small, manageable challenges with support build resilience. The child who learns to tolerate minor frustrations develops capacity for bigger challenges.

Technology in Crisis Management

Technology increasingly supports crisis intervention and safety management.

Crisis apps provide in-the-moment support. Safety planning apps store coping strategies, contacts, and reasons for living. Mood tracking apps identify patterns predicting crisis. Skill apps guide through DBT techniques during distress.

But technology isn't magic. Apps supplement but don't replace human connection. The suicidal teenager needs real relationships, not just smartphone interventions.

Electronic health records improve crisis response. Shared crisis plans ensure consistency across shifts and settings. Alert systems flag high-risk patients. Data tracking identifies patterns invisible in single moments.

Telepsychiatry enables expert consultation during crisis. The rural hospital can connect with child psychiatrists during emergency. The residential facility can access specialized consultation. Technology expands expertise beyond geographic limits.

Real-World Crisis Challenges

Crisis intervention theory meets messy reality in practice. Perfect protocols encounter imperfect situations requiring flexibility and judgment.

Staffing shortages compromise ideal responses. You might be managing multiple crises simultaneously. The perfect one-on-one de-escalation becomes impossible with three children escalating and two staff. Prioritize safety while acknowledging limitations.

Secondary trauma affects crisis responders. Repeated exposure to children's trauma, violence, and suicidality takes a toll. Your own trauma responses might activate during crises. Regular supervision, debriefing, and self-care aren't luxuries but necessities for sustained crisis work.

System failures complicate crisis management. The child who needs hospitalization but no beds exist. The family that needs intensive services but insurance denies. The school that needs support but lacks resources. Working within broken systems while maintaining hope challenges everyone.

Cultural considerations influence crisis expression and intervention. Some cultures express distress somatically. Others view mental health crises as spiritual problems. Direct eye contact might be disrespectful, not defiant. Understanding cultural context prevents misinterpretation and improves intervention.

Post-Crisis Recovery

What happens after crisis matters as much as the intervention itself. Post-crisis recovery determines whether crises become learning experiences or traumatic memories.

Immediate post-crisis focuses on safety and stabilization. Check for injuries - physical and emotional. Provide comfort items. Allow rest. The exhausted child who just de-escalated from violence needs recovery time before processing.

Reunification with milieu requires planning. Other children witnessed or heard the crisis. They need reassurance and processing too. The aggressive child returning to unit needs supported re-integration, not isolation or judgment.

Debriefing should happen soon but not immediately. The child needs to be calm enough to think. Usually within 24 hours works best. Focus on understanding, not blame. "Help me understand what happened" opens dialogue better than "Why did you do that?"

Collaborative analysis identifies patterns. What triggered escalation? What helped or didn't? What could be different next time? The child who participates in analysis develops insight and agency.

Repair relationships damaged during crisis. The child who threatened peers needs supervised reconciliation. The teenager who destroyed property might help repair. Restoration matters more than punishment.

Crisis plan revision incorporates lessons learned. Maybe different warning signs emerged. Perhaps new coping strategies helped. Maybe family involvement needs adjustment. Each crisis provides data for better future response.

Celebrate successes within crisis. The child who usually restrains for hours but calmed in thirty minutes showed progress. The teenager who asked for help before attempting suicide demonstrated growth. Finding victories within crises maintains hope.

Building Crisis Resilience

The goal isn't eliminating crises but building capacity to weather them. Children who develop crisis resilience transform from victims of overwhelming emotions to agents of their own recovery.

Predictability reduces crisis frequency. When children know what to expect, anxiety decreases. Clear schedules, consistent responses, and reliable relationships prevent many crises.

Skill building provides tools for future crises. Every successfully managed crisis builds confidence. The child who learns to ride out panic attacks develops mastery. The teenager who survives suicidal urges gains strength.

Meaning-making transforms crisis into growth. Help children understand crises as responses to overwhelming situations, not character flaws. The narrative shifts from "I'm bad" to "I was overwhelmed and now I'm learning."

Community support sustains crisis recovery. Isolated children face higher crisis risk. Building connections - with family, peers, mentors - creates safety nets. The teenager with multiple supportive relationships has alternatives when one fails.

Essential Crisis Principles

Crisis intervention in pediatric psychiatric nursing requires courage, compassion, and clinical skill. You're managing immediate danger while preserving therapeutic relationships, teaching skills while ensuring safety, and holding hope while acknowledging real risk.

Stay regulated yourself. Your calm nervous system is your most powerful tool. If you're escalated, you escalate others. Take breaks, seek supervision, and practice your own coping skills.

Respect dignity within safety. Yes, safety comes first, but how you ensure safety matters. The child restrained respectfully experiences different trauma than one restrained punitively.

Learn from every crisis. Each escalation teaches something - about triggers, effective interventions, system gaps. Without learning, crises simply repeat.

Maintain hope. The child in crisis today might be tomorrow's peer counselor. The teenager attempting suicide might become a suicide prevention advocate. Crisis doesn't define destiny.

Most importantly, recognize that crisis intervention is relationship intervention. The trust built through respectful crisis management enables future therapeutic work. The child who experiences you as helpful during their worst moment will trust you with their healing journey.

That fifteen-year-old from the opening? You entered the quiet room calmly, sat on the floor at safe distance, and said simply, "This is really hard." She screamed more, then gradually quieted. You offered her weighted blanket - she threw it but then retrieved it. An hour later, she was talking about her father, crying genuine grief rather than traumatic overwhelm. No restraints, no medication, no security. Just presence, patience, and professional skill.

Crisis intervention isn't about control - it's about connection. When you connect with a child in crisis, you offer them what they need most: someone who sees their pain, stays present despite it, and believes in their capacity to survive it. That's the heart of pediatric psychiatric nursing - meeting children in their darkest moments with skill, compassion, and unshakeable faith in their resilience.

Chapter 10: Trauma-Informed Care and Complex Trauma

When 8-year-old Marcus arrived at the pediatric clinic for his annual checkup, his foster mother mentioned he'd been having nightmares and "acting out" at school. During the examination, Marcus flinched when the nurse reached to check his blood pressure and asked repeatedly if the procedures would hurt. His chart showed this was his fourth placement in two years.

What Marcus's healthcare team didn't initially realize was that his behaviors weren't defiance or attention-seeking—they were the predictable responses of a developing brain and nervous system shaped by chronic trauma and disrupted attachments. Understanding this difference transforms how we approach care for children like Marcus and thousands of others who've experienced significant adversity.

Trauma isn't just something that happens to children—it fundamentally changes how their brains develop, how they view the world, and how they respond to stress. For pediatric nurses, recognizing trauma's impact and implementing trauma-informed approaches can mean the difference between triggering additional harm and becoming part of a child's healing journey.

Adverse Childhood Experiences and Developmental Trauma

The groundbreaking Adverse Childhood Experiences (ACEs) study, conducted by the Centers for Disease Control and Prevention and Kaiser Permanente, revealed startling connections between childhood adversity and lifelong health outcomes. This research showed that traumatic experiences during childhood don't just affect

123

emotional wellbeing—they literally reshape brain architecture and influence physical health for decades to come.

ACEs include ten categories of childhood adversity:

Abuse:

- Physical abuse
- Sexual abuse
- Emotional abuse

Neglect:

- Physical neglect
- Emotional neglect

Household Dysfunction:

- Mother treated violently
- Household substance abuse
- Mental illness in household
- Parental separation or divorce
- Incarcerated family member

The study's findings were sobering. Nearly 64% of adults reported having at least one ACE, while 12.6% experienced four or more ACEs. Children with higher ACE scores showed dramatically increased risks for depression, suicide attempts, substance abuse, heart disease, cancer, and premature death.

But here's what makes this particularly relevant for pediatric nurses: **ACEs don't affect all children equally**. The timing of trauma, the child's developmental stage, available support systems, and individual resilience factors all influence outcomes. A 3-year-old experiencing parental divorce will be affected differently than a 15-year-old facing the same situation.

Developmental trauma occurs when children experience chronic, prolonged exposure to traumatic events during critical developmental periods. Unlike single-incident trauma (like a car accident), developmental trauma typically involves repeated experiences of fear, helplessness, and threat within the child's caregiving system.

Children experiencing developmental trauma often struggle with:

- **Attachment disruptions**: Difficulty forming trusting relationships
- **Self-regulation problems**: Challenges managing emotions and behaviors
- **Self-concept issues**: Negative beliefs about themselves and their worth
- **Cognitive difficulties**: Problems with attention, learning, and memory
- **Behavioral challenges**: Aggression, withdrawal, or risky behaviors

Think about Sarah, a 12-year-old whose mother has untreated bipolar disorder. Sarah never knows if mom will be loving and attentive or angry and unpredictable. She's learned to scan her mother's face for signs of danger, to stay hypervigilant, and to take care of herself when mom can't. These survival skills helped Sarah cope at home, but they create problems at school where teachers interpret her vigilance as defiance and her self-reliance as stubbornness.

SAMHSA's Six Principles of Trauma-Informed Care

The Substance Abuse and Mental Health Services Administration (SAMHSA) developed six fundamental principles that guide trauma-informed approaches across all settings. These principles help organizations and individuals understand how to create environments that promote healing rather than re-traumatization.

Principle 1: Safety Physical and psychological safety forms the foundation of trauma-informed care. For children who've experienced trauma, feeling unsafe triggers their survival responses and makes healing impossible.

Physical safety includes:

- Clean, well-lit environments
- Clear sight lines and escape routes
- Comfortable temperature and seating
- Absence of potential weapons or triggers

Psychological safety involves:

- Predictable routines and clear expectations
- Respectful, non-judgmental interactions
- Confidentiality protections
- Cultural sensitivity and acceptance

In practice, this might mean letting a child know exactly what will happen during a medical procedure, allowing them to keep a comfort item during treatment, or positioning yourself at their eye level rather than looming over them.

Principle 2: Trustworthiness and Transparency Building trust requires consistent, honest communication and transparent operations. Children who've experienced trauma often have their trust repeatedly violated, making them hyperaware of inconsistencies or deception.

Trustworthiness means:

- Following through on promises, no matter how small
- Admitting when you don't know something
- Being honest about potential discomfort or challenges
- Maintaining consistent boundaries and expectations

Transparency involves:

- Explaining your role and the purpose of interactions
- Sharing information about policies and procedures
- Being open about treatment options and limitations
- Including children in age-appropriate decision-making

Principle 3: Peer Support Mutual self-help provides a key vehicle for healing from trauma. While this principle primarily applies to adult services, it's adapted for children through:

- Support groups for children with similar experiences
- Mentorship programs pairing children with older youth
- Family support groups connecting parents and caregivers
- Peer navigation services in healthcare settings

Principle 4: Collaboration and Mutuality Trauma-informed organizations recognize that healing happens in relationship and community. Everyone has a role to play in creating healing environments.

For pediatric settings, collaboration means:

- Partnering with children and families in treatment planning
- Including children's voices in program development
- Working across disciplines and agencies
- Sharing power and decision-making appropriately

This doesn't mean children make all decisions about their care, but it does mean their preferences, concerns, and ideas are valued and incorporated whenever possible.

Principle 5: Empowerment, Voice, and Choice Trauma often involves powerlessness and loss of control. Trauma-informed care actively works to restore a sense of agency and empowerment.

In pediatric settings, this includes:

- Offering choices whenever possible (which arm for the blood draw, sitting or lying down for the exam)

- Teaching children about their bodies and health
- Building on existing strengths and skills
- Supporting children's autonomy development
- Celebrating progress and achievements

Principle 6: Cultural, Historical, and Gender Issues Trauma-informed organizations actively move past cultural stereotypes and biases, offer healing approaches that are responsive to racial, ethnic, and cultural backgrounds, and recognize the impact of historical trauma.

This principle acknowledges that:

- Different cultures have varying approaches to healing and help-seeking
- Historical traumas (slavery, genocide, forced migration) affect entire communities across generations
- Gender identity and expression influence trauma experiences
- Language barriers can increase trauma and complicate treatment
- Religious and spiritual beliefs may be important resources for healing

Evidence-Based Trauma Interventions

While trauma's effects can be devastating, research has identified several highly effective interventions for helping children heal. These evidence-based treatments have been rigorously tested and shown to reduce trauma symptoms and improve functioning.

Trauma-Focused Cognitive Behavioral Therapy (TF-CBT)

TF-CBT is considered the gold standard for treating children aged 3-18 who've experienced trauma. This approach combines cognitive-behavioral techniques with trauma-sensitive interventions, always including a caregiver component.

The TF-CBT model includes several key components:

- **Psychoeducation**: Teaching children and caregivers about trauma's effects
- **Relaxation skills**: Building tools for managing anxiety and stress
- **Affective expression and modulation**: Learning to identify and regulate emotions
- **Cognitive coping**: Addressing unhelpful thoughts and beliefs
- **Trauma narrative**: Gradually processing the traumatic experience
- **In vivo mastery**: Facing trauma reminders in safe ways
- **Conjoint child-parent sessions**: Rebuilding trust and communication
- **Enhancing safety**: Developing protection plans

Research shows TF-CBT effectively reduces PTSD symptoms, depression, anxiety, and behavioral problems while improving children's overall functioning. The treatment typically lasts 12-20 sessions and can be adapted for individual children's needs.

Consider Maria, a 10-year-old who witnessed domestic violence between her parents. In TF-CBT, she learned relaxation breathing to manage her anxiety, identified thinking patterns that made her feel responsible for the violence, and gradually told her story in a safe, supportive environment. Her mother participated throughout, learning how to support Maria's healing and address her own trauma responses.

Child-Parent Psychotherapy (CPP)

CPP is specifically designed for children aged 0-5 who've experienced trauma and focuses on repairing the parent-child relationship. Young children can't process trauma through talk therapy alone—they need their relationships to be the vehicle for healing.

CPP addresses:

- **Attachment disruptions** caused by trauma
- **Developmental regression** common after traumatic experiences
- **Behavioral problems** that interfere with daily functioning
- **Parent-child interaction patterns** that may maintain trauma symptoms

The intervention is relationship-based, culturally responsive, and typically lasts 12-18 months. Therapists work with parent-child dyads to strengthen their bond, improve communication, and develop new patterns of interaction.

Attachment, Regulation, and Competency (ARC)

ARC is a flexible intervention framework designed for children and adolescents who've experienced complex trauma. Rather than following a rigid protocol, ARC provides a roadmap for addressing the three key areas affected by complex trauma:

Attachment: Building safe, stable relationships *Regulation:* Developing skills for managing emotions, behaviors, and thoughts *Competency:* Fostering children's sense of mastery and self-efficacy

ARC can be implemented in various settings—residential treatment, outpatient therapy, schools, or child welfare agencies. The approach emphasizes building on children's existing strengths while addressing trauma's impact on their development.

Other Evidence-Based Interventions

Several other approaches show strong research support:

- **Eye Movement Desensitization and Reprocessing (EMDR)**: Particularly effective for older children and adolescents with PTSD

- **Cognitive Behavioral Intervention for Trauma in Schools (CBITS)**: Group-based intervention delivered in school settings
- **Bounce Back**: A school-based program for children exposed to traumatic events
- **Structured Psychotherapy for Adolescents Responding to Chronic Stress (SPARCS)**: For adolescents with complex trauma histories

Special Populations and Unique Considerations

Certain groups of children face heightened trauma exposure and require specialized approaches. Understanding these populations' unique needs helps ensure culturally responsive, effective care.

Refugee and Immigrant Children

Children who've fled their home countries often carry multiple layers of trauma. Pre-migration trauma might include war exposure, violence, or persecution. Migration itself can be traumatic, involving dangerous journeys, family separation, or detention. Post-migration stress includes language barriers, discrimination, poverty, and cultural adjustment challenges.

These children may present with:

- **Somatic symptoms**: Headaches, stomachaches, or other physical complaints
- **Sleep disturbances**: Nightmares, insomnia, or fear of sleeping alone
- **School difficulties**: Problems concentrating, learning English, or adjusting to new educational systems
- **Family stress**: Role reversals where children translate or navigate systems for parents
- **Identity confusion**: Struggling to balance home culture with new environment

Healthcare providers working with refugee children should:

- Use professional interpreters, never children or family members
- Understand that symptoms may be normal responses to abnormal situations
- Connect families with culturally specific services and supports
- Be aware of potential triggers (uniforms, medical procedures that resemble torture)
- Recognize that healing often occurs within cultural and community contexts

Child Trafficking Victims

Human trafficking affects an estimated 300,000 American children annually, though exact numbers are difficult to determine due to the hidden nature of these crimes. Trafficked children experience severe trauma including physical and sexual abuse, psychological manipulation, social isolation, and exposure to violence.

These children often don't self-identify as victims and may be suspicious of helping professionals. They might:

- Have been taught to distrust law enforcement and healthcare providers
- Fear deportation if they're undocumented immigrants
- Experience trauma bonds with traffickers who provided basic needs
- Have untreated medical conditions or injuries
- Show signs of malnutrition, sleep deprivation, or substance use

Healthcare providers must be trained to recognize trafficking indicators and respond appropriately. This includes understanding mandatory reporting requirements, accessing specialized services, and providing trauma-informed care that doesn't re-victimize children.

Child Abuse Survivors

Children who've experienced abuse within their families face unique challenges because their trauma occurred within their primary attachment relationships. These children often struggle with:

- **Attachment disorganization**: Simultaneous fear and need for closeness
- **Self-blame**: Believing they caused or deserved the abuse
- **Hypervigilance**: Constantly scanning for danger signals
- **Developmental delays**: Due to chronic stress and neglect
- **Behavioral extremes**: Either overly compliant or aggressive

Working with abuse survivors requires particular sensitivity to power dynamics. These children have learned that adults can be dangerous, so building trust takes time and consistency. They may test boundaries repeatedly or alternate between clinging and pushing away.

Trauma Screening and Assessment Tools

Effective trauma-informed care begins with appropriate screening and assessment. Various tools help identify children who've experienced trauma and assess its impact on their functioning.

Universal Screening Tools

ACE Questionnaire: Screens for ten categories of childhood adversity *Pediatric ACEs and Related Life-events Screener (PEARLS):* Trauma screening tool for children ages 0-21 *BRFSS ACE Module:* Population-level screening for ACEs prevalence

Trauma-Specific Assessment Tools

Clinician-Administered PTSD Scale for Children and Adolescents (CAPS-CA): Gold standard diagnostic interview for PTSD *Childhood Trauma Questionnaire (CTQ):* Assesses five types of maltreatment *Trauma Symptom Checklist for Children (TSCC):* Measures trauma symptoms in children ages 8-16 *Child PTSD*

Symptom Scale (CPSS): Self-report measure for children and adolescents

Caregiver and Family Assessment Tools

Parental Stress Scale: Assesses stress related to parenting *Adult-Adolescent Parenting Inventory (AAPI):* Evaluates parenting attitudes and practices *Family Assessment Device (FAD):* Measures family functioning across multiple dimensions

Considerations for Trauma Screening

Trauma screening must be conducted thoughtfully to avoid re-traumatization. Best practices include:

- Creating safe, private environments for screening
- Explaining the purpose and process clearly
- Allowing children to control the pace of disclosure
- Having safety planning resources readily available
- Following up positive screens with appropriate referrals
- Training all staff on trauma-informed screening approaches

Environmental Factors and Healing Spaces

The physical environment plays a crucial role in supporting or hindering healing from trauma. Trauma-informed environments are designed to promote safety, comfort, and empowerment.

Physical Environment Considerations

Lighting: Natural light when possible, soft artificial lighting, avoiding harsh fluorescents *Colors:* Calming, warm colors rather than institutional white or bright primary colors *Furniture:* Comfortable, moveable seating that allows for personal space preferences *Noise:* Minimizing loud, unexpected sounds that might trigger startle responses *Space:* Providing both private areas and open, welcoming common spaces

Sensory Considerations

Children with trauma histories often have heightened sensory sensitivities. Healing environments consider:

- Texture variety in furniture and materials
- Pleasant, mild scents (avoiding strong perfumes or cleaners)
- Background music or sound machines for masking
- Fidget toys or stress balls available
- Weighted blankets or other calming sensory tools

Cultural Elements

Trauma-informed environments reflect the communities they serve:

- Artwork and decorations representing diverse cultures
- Materials available in multiple languages
- Space for cultural or religious practices
- Foods and beverages that feel welcoming to different groups

Safety and Security Features

While maintaining a welcoming atmosphere, trauma-informed environments also prioritize safety:

- Clear sight lines and multiple exit routes
- Secure areas for storing personal belongings
- Emergency communication systems
- Staff trained in de-escalation techniques
- Clear policies about confidentiality and mandatory reporting

Self-Care Strategies for Providers

Working with traumatized children affects healthcare providers profoundly. Secondary trauma, also called vicarious trauma, occurs when professionals absorb the emotional residue of working with trauma survivors. Without proper self-care, providers risk burnout, compassion fatigue, and their own trauma symptoms.

Recognizing Secondary Trauma

Signs of secondary trauma include:

- Intrusive thoughts about clients' experiences
- Nightmares or sleep disturbances
- Emotional numbing or detachment
- Increased cynicism or hopelessness
- Physical symptoms like headaches or digestive issues
- Avoiding certain types of cases or clients
- Relationship difficulties

Individual Self-Care Strategies

Physical self-care:

- Regular exercise and movement
- Adequate sleep and nutrition
- Medical and dental care
- Relaxation and stress reduction techniques

Emotional self-care:

- Personal therapy or counseling
- Journaling or creative expression
- Spiritual practices or meditation
- Maintaining friendships and social connections

Professional self-care:

- Continuing education and skill development
- Professional supervision or consultation
- Setting appropriate boundaries
- Taking vacation time and breaks

Organizational Self-Care Support

Healthcare organizations have responsibility for supporting staff wellbeing:

- Providing regular supervision and support
- Offering employee assistance programs
- Creating reasonable caseloads and expectations
- Training staff in trauma-informed approaches
- Promoting work-life balance
- Addressing organizational trauma and stress

Building Resilience

Resilience isn't just about bouncing back from adversity—it's about growing stronger through challenges. Healthcare providers can build resilience through:

- Developing a sense of purpose and meaning in work
- Building strong professional and personal relationships
- Maintaining hope and optimism
- Practicing gratitude and mindfulness
- Learning from difficult experiences
- Staying connected to personal values and beliefs

Implementation Challenges and Solutions

Implementing trauma-informed care isn't always straightforward. Healthcare organizations face various challenges in creating truly trauma-informed environments.

Common Implementation Challenges

Limited resources: Trauma-informed care requires training, supervision, and sometimes environmental modifications *Staff resistance:* Some providers may resist changing established practices *Time constraints:* Building trust and providing trauma-informed care takes time *Competing priorities:* Healthcare settings have multiple demands and requirements *Lack of trauma training:* Many providers haven't received adequate trauma education

Solutions and Strategies

Start with leadership commitment: Trauma-informed care must be supported at all organizational levels *Provide comprehensive training:* All staff need basic trauma awareness, with specialized training for direct care providers *Create policies and procedures:* Formalize trauma-informed approaches in organizational protocols *Use data to drive improvement:* Track outcomes and adjust approaches based on results *Build partnerships:* Collaborate with trauma specialists and community organizations

Measuring Success

Trauma-informed care implementation can be measured through:

- Reduced use of restraints and seclusion
- Decreased staff turnover and burnout
- Improved patient satisfaction scores
- Better treatment engagement and outcomes
- Reduced emergency department visits and crisis interventions

Working with Families in Trauma-Informed Ways

Families are often the key to children's healing from trauma, but families may also be struggling with their own trauma responses. Trauma-informed care with families requires balancing support with appropriate boundaries.

Understanding Family Trauma

Trauma often affects entire family systems, not just individual children. Parents may:

- Have their own trauma histories that are triggered by their child's experiences
- Feel guilt, shame, or responsibility for their child's trauma
- Struggle with their own mental health or substance use issues

- Face practical challenges like housing instability or financial stress
- Experience secondary trauma from learning about their child's experiences

Family-Centered Trauma-Informed Approaches

Engage families as partners: Recognize parents and caregivers as experts on their children *Provide psychoeducation:* Help families understand trauma's effects and the healing process *Build on family strengths:* Identify and reinforce positive family patterns and resources *Address practical needs:* Help families access housing, food, transportation, and other basic needs *Support cultural practices:* Incorporate families' cultural and spiritual approaches to healing *Connect with supports:* Link families to peer support groups and community resources

Special Considerations for Different Age Groups

Trauma affects children differently depending on their developmental stage. Trauma-informed care must be adapted to match children's cognitive, emotional, and social development.

Infants and Toddlers (0-3 years)

Very young children can't verbally process traumatic experiences, but trauma profoundly affects their developing brains and attachment relationships. Trauma-informed care for this age group focuses on:

- Supporting caregiver-infant relationships
- Addressing feeding, sleeping, and other routine disruptions
- Providing sensory regulation support
- Creating predictable, soothing environments
- Working with caregivers to understand infant cues and needs

Preschoolers (3-5 years)

Preschool children have limited language for describing their experiences and often express trauma through play and behavior. They may:

- Engage in repetitive play themes related to trauma
- Show increased aggression or withdrawal
- Experience regression in developmental milestones
- Have difficulty separating from caregivers
- Struggle with emotional regulation

Trauma-informed approaches include:

- Using play therapy techniques
- Helping children develop feeling words and coping skills
- Working closely with caregivers to support consistent routines
- Addressing sleep and behavioral difficulties
- Providing patient, nurturing interactions

School-Age Children (6-11 years)

School-age children can better understand and articulate their experiences but still need concrete, age-appropriate explanations. They may experience:

- Academic difficulties and school avoidance
- Peer relationship problems
- Somatic complaints (headaches, stomachaches)
- Increased anxiety and worry
- Difficulty concentrating

Trauma-informed care includes:

- Collaborating with schools to support academic success
- Teaching concrete coping skills and strategies
- Addressing physical symptoms with appropriate medical care
- Building peer relationships and social skills

- Involving children in age-appropriate treatment planning

Adolescents (12-18 years)

Teenagers face unique challenges because trauma occurs during a time of identity formation and increased independence. They may:

- Engage in risky behaviors like substance use or self-harm
- Experience relationship difficulties and trust issues
- Struggle with self-image and identity
- Show increased depression and anxiety
- Have difficulty planning for the future

Trauma-informed approaches must:

- Balance autonomy with appropriate support and structure
- Address identity and self-esteem issues
- Teach healthy relationship skills
- Support future planning and goal-setting
- Involve adolescents as active partners in treatment

The Future of Trauma-Informed Care

The field of trauma-informed care continues to evolve as research reveals new understanding about trauma's effects and effective interventions. Several emerging trends are shaping the future of trauma-informed approaches.

Precision Medicine Approaches

Research is beginning to identify how genetic factors influence trauma responses and treatment effectiveness. In the future, providers may be able to use genetic information to:

- Predict which children are most vulnerable to trauma effects
- Tailor interventions to individual genetic profiles
- Identify children who may respond better to specific medications

141

- Develop personalized prevention strategies

Technology Integration

Technology offers new opportunities for delivering trauma-informed care:

- Virtual reality exposure therapy for treating PTSD
- Mobile apps for teaching coping skills and emotion regulation
- Telehealth services for reaching underserved populations
- Biometric monitoring to track stress responses and recovery
- Online training platforms for educating providers

Community-Based Approaches

There's growing recognition that healing from trauma requires community-wide responses:

- Trauma-informed schools that create healing environments for all students
- Community resilience initiatives that address historical and collective trauma
- Faith-based organizations providing culturally responsive healing approaches
- Peer support networks connecting trauma survivors and families

Prevention Focus

While treatment remains important, there's increasing emphasis on preventing trauma from occurring:

- Home visiting programs that support new families
- Community violence prevention initiatives
- Economic policies that reduce family stress and instability
- Educational programs that build resilience skills

- Social policies that address structural factors contributing to trauma

Bringing It All Together

Trauma-informed care represents a fundamental shift from asking "What's wrong with you?" to asking "What happened to you?" This simple change in perspective can transform how we understand and respond to children's behavioral and emotional challenges.

For pediatric nurses, implementing trauma-informed care means:

- Screening for trauma exposure and symptoms
- Creating safe, welcoming environments
- Building trusting relationships with children and families
- Using evidence-based interventions when appropriate
- Collaborating with trauma specialists and community resources
- Taking care of yourself to prevent secondary trauma

But trauma-informed care isn't just about individual interactions—it's about transforming entire systems to be more responsive to trauma's effects. This requires commitment from leadership, comprehensive staff training, policy changes, and ongoing quality improvement efforts.

The children we serve have shown tremendous strength and resilience in surviving traumatic experiences. Our role is to create conditions that support their natural healing processes while providing evidence-based interventions to address trauma's effects. When we get this right, we don't just treat symptoms—we help children reclaim their sense of safety, rebuild their capacity for trust, and develop the skills they need to thrive.

Marcus, the 8-year-old boy we met at the beginning of this chapter, is thriving now. His healthcare team learned to recognize his hypervigilance as a trauma response rather than defiance. They gave him choices whenever possible, explained procedures in advance, and worked closely with his foster family to create consistency across settings. His foster parents participated in trauma-focused therapy, learning how to provide the patient, nurturing care Marcus needed to heal.

Most importantly, everyone involved in Marcus's care understood that his behaviors made perfect sense given what he'd experienced. This understanding allowed them to respond with compassion rather than frustration, support rather than punishment, and hope rather than despair. That's the power of trauma-informed care—it helps us see strength where others might see pathology, resilience where others might see damage, and hope where others might see hopelessness.

Chapter 11: Cultural Competency and Special Populations

Fifteen-year-old Aaliyah sat silently in the mental health clinic waiting room, her hijab perfectly arranged, her eyes downcast. Her mother had brought her after teachers reported she seemed "withdrawn and sad." But when the therapist suggested individual sessions, Aaliyah's mother firmly shook her head. "We keep family matters private," she explained. "What will people think?"

In the next room, 16-year-old Alex fidgeted nervously, wondering whether to tell the nurse practitioner about feelings of not fitting into their assigned gender. Last month, a friend was kicked out of their home for being transgender. Would this provider be safe? Could Alex risk being honest?

Meanwhile, 12-year-old Joaquín, who'd been in three foster homes in the past year, tested every boundary his new therapist set. He'd learned that adults promise things they don't keep, that "help" often hurts more than it helps, and that it's safer to push people away before they inevitably leave.

These three young people represent just a fraction of the diverse populations pediatric mental health providers encounter daily. Each brings unique cultural backgrounds, experiences of marginalization, and specific needs that require culturally responsive, affirming care approaches. Understanding how culture, identity, and social position influence mental health experiences isn't just about being politically correct—it's about providing effective, healing-centered care.

Cultural Competency Frameworks

Culture shapes everything about how we experience and express mental health challenges. It influences how families understand emotional distress, what help-seeking looks like, which treatments feel acceptable, and what recovery means. For pediatric mental health providers, cultural competency isn't optional—it's essential for providing effective care.

But cultural competency goes deeper than knowing about different ethnic foods or holiday traditions. It requires understanding how systems of power and privilege affect access to care, how historical trauma impacts entire communities, and how current discrimination shapes children's daily experiences.

The Cultural Competency Continuum

Organizations and individuals exist at different points along a cultural competency continuum:

Cultural Destructiveness: Practices that harm culturally diverse groups *Cultural Incapacity:* Well-intentioned but ineffective approaches that maintain disparities *Cultural Blindness:* "Colorblind" approaches that ignore cultural differences *Cultural Pre-competence:* Awareness of limitations and commitment to improvement *Cultural Competency:* Evidence-based practices that effectively serve diverse populations *Cultural Proficiency:* Advocacy for systemic change and cultural responsiveness

Most healthcare organizations fall somewhere in the middle of this continuum, with pockets of excellence alongside areas needing significant improvement.

Key Components of Cultural Competency

Cultural Awareness: Understanding your own cultural background and biases *Cultural Knowledge:* Learning about different cultural groups and their experiences *Cross-Cultural Skills:* Developing abilities to communicate and interact effectively across cultures *Cultural Encounters:* Seeking direct interactions with people from different cultural backgrounds *Cultural Desire:* Genuine motivation to become culturally competent

146

Beyond Individual Competency: Structural Approaches

While individual cultural competency remains important, research increasingly emphasizes the need for structural and organizational changes. This includes:

- Hiring diverse staff at all organizational levels
- Implementing policies that address bias and discrimination
- Using data to identify and eliminate disparities
- Creating inclusive physical environments
- Partnering with community organizations

Mental Health Disparities

Mental health disparities aren't accidents—they're the predictable result of systemic inequities that affect access to care, quality of services, and health outcomes. Understanding these disparities helps providers recognize why culturally responsive care is so crucial.

Prevalence Disparities

Different racial and ethnic groups show varying rates of mental health conditions:

- *American Indian/Alaska Native* youth have the highest rates of suicide (18.2 per 100,000)
- *Black* children are more likely to experience trauma but less likely to receive treatment
- *Latino* adolescents show high rates of depression but face significant treatment barriers
- *Asian American* youth often underutilize mental health services despite similar prevalence rates

Access and Quality Disparities

Even when children from diverse backgrounds access mental health services, they often receive lower quality care:

- Children of color are more likely to receive services in emergency departments rather than outpatient settings
- Treatment dropout rates are higher for racial and ethnic minority families
- Misdiagnosis rates are elevated for certain populations
- Culturally adapted interventions are rarely available

Contributing Factors

Several interrelated factors contribute to these disparities:

Structural Racism: Systemic policies and practices that disadvantage people of color *Provider Bias:* Conscious and unconscious stereotypes that affect clinical decision-making *Language Barriers:* Limited availability of services in languages other than English *Economic Factors:* Poverty, unemployment, and lack of insurance *Geographic Barriers:* Limited services in rural or underserved communities *Cultural Mistrust:* Historical and ongoing experiences of discrimination in healthcare

Population-Specific Approaches

While every child is unique, certain populations share common experiences that inform culturally responsive care approaches. Understanding these patterns helps providers offer more effective services while avoiding stereotyping individuals.

Racial and Ethnic Minorities

African American/Black Children and Families

African American families navigate unique stressors including ongoing racism, economic inequality, and historical trauma from slavery, segregation, and systemic exclusion. These factors influence mental health in complex ways.

Strengths and Resources:

- Strong extended family and kinship networks
- Religious and spiritual traditions that provide meaning and support
- Community resilience and collective coping strategies
- Cultural values emphasizing perseverance and strength

Challenges and Risk Factors:

- Higher exposure to community violence and trauma
- Disproportionate contact with child welfare and juvenile justice systems
- Educational disparities and school-to-prison pipeline effects
- Discrimination in healthcare settings

Culturally Responsive Approaches:

- Incorporate spirituality and faith-based supports when appropriate
- Address racism and discrimination as mental health stressors
- Build on family and community strengths
- Use culturally adapted interventions when available
- Collaborate with Black mental health professionals and community organizations

Consider Keisha, a 14-year-old Black girl who was referred for "aggressive behavior" after an altercation with a teacher. Rather than focusing solely on her behavior, a culturally competent provider would explore whether she'd experienced racial microaggressions at school, how her family talks about coping with racism, and what community supports might be available.

Latino/Hispanic Children and Families

Latino families represent diverse backgrounds including Mexican, Puerto Rican, Cuban, Central American, and South American origins. While sharing some common cultural values, each group has unique historical experiences and needs.

Strengths and Resources:

- Strong family orientation (*familismo*)
- Respect for authority and tradition (*respeto*)
- Religious and spiritual beliefs
- Bilingual abilities and cultural bridging skills

Challenges and Risk Factors:

- Immigration-related stress and trauma
- Language barriers in healthcare settings
- Economic marginalization and employment challenges
- Discrimination and anti-immigrant sentiment
- Intergenerational conflicts around cultural values

Culturally Responsive Approaches:

- Provide services in Spanish when needed
- Involve extended family in treatment planning
- Address immigration concerns and their mental health impacts
- Use *dichos* (sayings) and cultural metaphors in therapy
- Connect families with culturally specific community resources

Asian American and Pacific Islander Children and Families

Asian American and Pacific Islander (AAPI) populations include dozens of distinct ethnic groups with varying languages, cultures, and immigration experiences. Mental health stigma is often pronounced in many AAPI communities.

Strengths and Resources:

- Strong educational values and achievement orientation
- Extended family support systems
- Cultural practices promoting harmony and balance
- Resilience and adaptability

150

Challenges and Risk Factors:

- Mental health stigma and shame
- Pressure to achieve and maintain family honor
- Intergenerational conflicts around cultural values
- Language barriers and limited culturally appropriate services
- Model minority myth that obscures real needs

Culturally Responsive Approaches:

- Address stigma directly and normalize mental health treatment
- Include family members in culturally appropriate ways
- Use indirect communication styles when appropriate
- Incorporate cultural concepts of balance and harmony
- Provide psychoeducation about mental health in cultural context

Native American/American Indian Children and Families

Native American communities face unique challenges related to historical trauma, ongoing colonization effects, and cultural disruption. Each tribe has distinct cultural traditions and healing practices.

Strengths and Resources:

- Traditional healing practices and ceremonies
- Connection to land and nature
- Oral traditions and storytelling
- Extended family and tribal support systems

Challenges and Risk Factors:

- Historical trauma from genocide, boarding schools, and cultural suppression
- High rates of suicide, substance use, and trauma exposure
- Geographic isolation and limited services

- Poverty and limited economic opportunities
- Loss of cultural identity and practices

Culturally Responsive Approaches:

- Learn about specific tribal cultures and histories
- Incorporate traditional healing practices when appropriate
- Address historical trauma and its ongoing effects
- Connect families with tribal resources and supports
- Use circular rather than linear treatment approaches

LGBTQ+ Youth

LGBTQ+ young people face significant mental health challenges, with rates of depression, anxiety, and suicidal ideation far exceeding those of their heterosexual, cisgender peers. Creating affirming care environments can literally save lives.

Understanding Sexual Orientation and Gender Identity Development

Sexual orientation and gender identity typically develop during childhood and adolescence, though the process varies greatly among individuals. Key concepts include:

Sexual Orientation: Who someone is romantically or sexually attracted to *Gender Identity:* Someone's internal sense of being male, female, both, or neither *Gender Expression:* How someone presents their gender through clothing, behavior, voice, etc. *Cisgender:* When gender identity matches assigned sex at birth *Transgender:* When gender identity differs from assigned sex at birth

Mental Health Disparities

LGBTQ+ youth experience alarming rates of mental health challenges:

- *41% of LGBTQ+ youth* seriously considered attempting suicide in the past year
- *Transgender and nonbinary youth* are at especially high risk
- *Family rejection* increases suicide risk by 8 times
- *School bullying* affects 84% of LGBTQ+ students

Risk Factors

Several factors contribute to poor mental health outcomes:

- Family rejection or lack of acceptance
- Bullying and victimization at school
- Discrimination and harassment in community settings
- Internalized homophobia or transphobia
- Lack of LGBTQ+ affirming healthcare
- Social isolation and lack of peer support

Protective Factors

Research identifies several factors that protect LGBTQ+ youth:

- Family acceptance and support
- School policies that protect LGBTQ+ students
- Access to Gay-Straight Alliance groups
- LGBTQ+ affirming healthcare providers
- Connection to LGBTQ+ community and role models

Affirming Care Practices

Creating LGBTQ+ affirming environments involves both clinical practices and organizational policies:

Clinical Practices:

- Use chosen names and pronouns consistently
- Ask about sexual orientation and gender identity respectfully
- Understand developmental aspects of LGBTQ+ identity
- Address minority stress and discrimination

- Connect youth with LGBTQ+ affirming resources

Organizational Policies:

- Train all staff in LGBTQ+ cultural competency
- Update intake forms to be inclusive
- Create gender-neutral bathrooms when possible
- Display LGBTQ+ affirming symbols and materials
- Develop non-discrimination policies that include LGBTQ+ protections

Consider Jordan, a 16-year-old who recently came out as transgender to their school counselor. Jordan's parents are struggling to understand and haven't agreed to use their chosen name. An LGBTQ+ affirming provider would validate Jordan's identity, help them cope with family stress, and potentially facilitate family meetings to improve understanding and support.

Foster Care Youth

Approximately 400,000 children live in foster care on any given day, with many experiencing multiple placements and ongoing instability. These youth face extraordinary mental health challenges due to early trauma, family separation, and system involvement.

Unique Challenges

Foster youth experience multiple layers of adversity:

- *Original trauma* that led to removal from home
- *Separation trauma* from losing family connections
- *System trauma* from multiple placements and workers
- *Identity disruption* from lack of consistent caregiving
- *Educational disruption* from school changes
- *Aging out* challenges for older youth

Mental Health Needs

Foster youth show significantly higher rates of mental health conditions:

- *60% have behavioral or emotional problems*
- *30% have been diagnosed with ADHD*
- *25% have mood disorders*
- *Psychotropic medication use* is 5 times higher than other children

Systemic Challenges

Several system factors complicate mental health treatment:

- Consent issues when children are in state custody
- Frequent placement changes disrupting treatment
- Limited resources for specialized services
- Coordination challenges between multiple agencies
- Lack of trauma-informed approaches in many placements

Best Practices for Foster Youth

Effective mental health care for foster youth requires system-level approaches:

Clinical Practices:

- Comprehensive trauma screening and assessment
- Coordination with child welfare workers and attorneys
- Focus on building stability and trust
- Address grief and loss related to family separation
- Prepare youth for aging out of care

System Practices:

- Minimize placement disruptions
- Maintain connections to siblings and important adults
- Ensure educational stability
- Provide life skills training for older youth

- Support successful transitions to adulthood

Resource Families and Therapeutic Parenting

Foster and kinship caregivers need specialized training and support to address the complex needs of children who've experienced trauma. Therapeutic parenting approaches help caregivers:

- Understand trauma's effects on behavior and development
- Use trauma-informed discipline strategies
- Build trust and attachment with children
- Advocate for appropriate services and supports
- Take care of themselves to prevent caregiver burnout

Justice-Involved Youth

Young people involved in the juvenile justice system have extremely high rates of mental health conditions, often stemming from trauma, poverty, and systemic inequities. Rather than receiving treatment, many youth receive punishment that worsens their conditions.

Mental Health Prevalence

Justice-involved youth show alarming rates of mental health conditions:

- *70% meet criteria* for at least one mental health condition
- *20% have serious mental illness*
- *Trauma exposure* affects 90% of detained youth
- *Substance use disorders* are common among older adolescents

Pathways to System Involvement

Several factors contribute to youth justice involvement:

- Untreated mental health conditions leading to behavioral problems
- School suspension and expulsion pushing youth out of education
- Trauma responses misinterpreted as defiance or aggression
- Poverty and lack of community resources
- Racial bias in policing and judicial decision-making

Challenges in Justice Settings

Mental health treatment in juvenile justice settings faces multiple barriers:

- Punitive rather than therapeutic environment
- Limited trained mental health staff
- Use of isolation and restraints that worsen trauma
- Inadequate screening and assessment
- Lack of continuity between detention and community care

Therapeutic Justice Approaches

Progressive jurisdictions are implementing therapeutic justice models:

- *Mental Health Courts* that divert youth to treatment rather than detention
- *Trauma-informed detention* facilities that prioritize healing over punishment
- *Community-based alternatives* that keep youth at home while providing intensive services
- *Restorative justice* approaches that focus on repairing harm rather than punishment

Homeless and Runaway Youth

An estimated 4.2 million youth experience homelessness each year, including those who are unaccompanied, living in unstable housing, or couch-surfing with friends or acquaintances. These youth face extraordinary mental health challenges while having limited access to services.

Pathways to Homelessness

Youth become homeless for various reasons:

- Family conflict and rejection, particularly for LGBTQ+ youth
- Physical, sexual, or emotional abuse at home
- Aging out of foster care without support
- Mental health or substance use problems
- Economic hardship affecting entire families
- Natural disasters or other traumatic events

Mental Health Challenges

Homeless youth experience high rates of mental health conditions:

- *Depression and anxiety* affect the majority of homeless youth
- *PTSD* is common due to trauma exposure
- *Substance use* often develops as a coping mechanism
- *Suicidal ideation* rates are significantly elevated
- *Self-harm behaviors* are more common than in housed youth

Barriers to Care

Multiple factors prevent homeless youth from accessing mental health services:

- Lack of insurance or identification documents
- No permanent address for appointments
- Transportation challenges
- Mistrust of helping systems
- Competing survival needs (food, shelter, safety)
- Age restrictions that exclude older adolescents from youth services

Best Practices for Homeless Youth

Effective services for homeless youth use low-barrier, youth-centered approaches:

Service Approaches:

- Meet youth where they are (literally and figuratively)
- Provide basic needs before addressing mental health
- Use harm reduction rather than abstinence-only approaches
- Build trust through consistent, non-judgmental relationships
- Address practical needs alongside mental health treatment

Program Components:

- Drop-in centers that provide immediate support
- Transitional living programs with supportive services
- Rapid rehousing assistance
- Job training and educational support
- Healthcare and mental health services
- Life skills development

Consider Maria, a 17-year-old who's been living on the streets for six months after her family rejected her for being lesbian. She's struggling with depression and using alcohol to cope but won't access traditional mental health services because she fears being forced back to her family. A youth-centered program would meet Maria's immediate needs for safety and shelter while building trust that might eventually lead to mental health treatment.

Cultural Assessment and Intervention Strategies

Providing culturally responsive mental health care requires systematic approaches to assessment and intervention that consider cultural factors throughout the treatment process.

Cultural Assessment Components

Comprehensive cultural assessment includes:

Cultural Identity:

- Ethnic and racial background
- Language preferences and fluency
- Religious or spiritual beliefs
- Sexual orientation and gender identity
- Socioeconomic status and experiences

Cultural Explanations:

- How the family understands the problem
- Traditional healing practices or remedies tried
- Spiritual or religious explanations for distress
- Cultural stigma or shame associated with mental health

Cultural Factors Related to Environment:

- Level of social support from cultural community
- Experiences of discrimination or prejudice
- Acculturation stress and cultural conflicts
- Access to culturally appropriate services

Cultural Features of Relationship:

- Power dynamics and authority relationships
- Communication styles and preferences
- Role of family in decision-making
- Gender role expectations

Culturally Adapted Interventions

While evidence-based treatments form the foundation of effective care, many have been developed and tested primarily with white, middle-class populations. Cultural adaptations modify these interventions to better fit diverse populations.

160

Types of cultural adaptations include:

Surface Adaptations:

- Translating materials into different languages
- Using culturally relevant examples and metaphors
- Including diverse images in treatment materials
- Matching clients with providers from similar backgrounds

Deep Structure Adaptations:

- Modifying treatment goals to fit cultural values
- Changing intervention techniques to match cultural preferences
- Incorporating traditional healing practices
- Addressing cultural factors that contribute to mental health problems

Examples of Culturally Adapted Treatments

Cuento Therapy: Uses traditional Latino folktales to teach coping skills and cultural values *Multisystemic Therapy for Child Abuse and Neglect:* Adapts MST for diverse families by incorporating cultural strengths *Trauma-Focused CBT:* Cultural adaptations address specific trauma types (war, persecution) and incorporate cultural healing practices

Building Cultural Bridges in Healthcare Settings

Creating culturally responsive healthcare environments requires attention to both interpersonal interactions and organizational structures.

Communication Across Cultures

Effective cross-cultural communication requires understanding different communication styles:

Direct vs. Indirect Communication: Some cultures value direct, explicit communication while others rely on context, nonverbal cues, and implied meanings.

Individual vs. Collective Decision-Making: Western mental health emphasizes individual autonomy, but many cultures prioritize family or community input in important decisions.

High-Context vs. Low-Context Cultures: High-context cultures rely heavily on situational factors and relationships, while low-context cultures focus on explicit verbal information.

Working with Interpreters

When language barriers exist, professional interpreters are essential for effective care:

Best Practices:

- Use professional interpreters, never family members or children
- Brief interpreters on mental health terminology beforehand
- Speak directly to the client, not the interpreter
- Ask interpreters to interpret everything said
- Debrief with interpreters after sessions when appropriate

Avoiding Common Mistakes:

- Don't assume family members can interpret accurately
- Don't use children as interpreters for their parents
- Don't rely on bilingual staff who aren't trained interpreters
- Don't skip interpretation for "simple" conversations

Addressing Bias and Microaggressions

Healthcare providers must examine their own biases and work to eliminate microaggressions—subtle forms of discrimination that communicate bias or prejudice.

Common Healthcare Microaggressions:

- Assuming someone's immigration status based on appearance
- Making assumptions about family structures or relationships
- Using incorrect names or pronouns
- Dismissing cultural explanations for mental health symptoms
- Showing surprise when people of color are educated or articulate

Strategies for Interrupting Bias:

- Regular self-examination and bias training
- Seeking feedback from diverse colleagues and community members
- Using structured decision-making tools to reduce bias
- Creating accountable systems for addressing bias when it occurs

Community Partnerships and Resources

Effective mental health care for diverse populations requires partnerships with community organizations that understand and serve specific cultural groups.

Types of Community Partners

Faith-Based Organizations: Many families turn first to religious leaders for help with mental health concerns. Partnering with faith communities can increase access and reduce stigma.

Cultural Organizations: Community centers, cultural associations, and ethnic media can help reach families and provide culturally grounded support.

Schools: Educational settings are often the first place mental health concerns are identified, making school partnerships essential.

Community Health Centers: Federally Qualified Health Centers and other community-based organizations often serve diverse populations and can be important referral sources.

Advocacy and Social Justice

Cultural competency in mental health must go beyond individual clinical interactions to address systemic factors that contribute to disparities.

Individual Advocacy:

- Helping families navigate complex healthcare systems
- Advocating for appropriate services and accommodations
- Addressing discrimination when it occurs
- Supporting families in educational and legal settings

Systems Advocacy:

- Working to eliminate discriminatory policies and practices
- Advocating for increased funding for culturally appropriate services
- Supporting policy changes that address social determinants of health
- Participating in community coalitions working for health equity

Building Your Cultural Competency Toolkit

Developing cultural competency is a lifelong journey that requires ongoing learning and self-reflection. Key strategies include:

Continuous Learning:

- Attending cultural competency training regularly
- Learning about communities you serve
- Reading literature by and about diverse populations
- Staying current on disparities research

164

Self-Reflection:

- Examining your own cultural background and biases
- Seeking feedback about your cross-cultural interactions
- Processing challenging cases with culturally competent supervisors
- Engaging in personal therapy to address your own biases and triggers

Skill Development:

- Learning basic phrases in languages spoken by clients
- Practicing cultural assessment techniques
- Developing cultural formulation skills
- Building comfort with difficult conversations about bias and discrimination

Relationship Building:

- Developing relationships with diverse community leaders
- Participating in cultural events and community activities
- Building a network of culturally competent colleagues
- Creating mentoring relationships with providers from different backgrounds

Technology and Cultural Responsiveness

Technology offers new opportunities for increasing access to culturally responsive mental health services, but it also creates new challenges that must be addressed.

Advantages of Technology

Increased Access:

- Telehealth can reach geographically isolated populations
- Online services can connect people with culturally matched providers

- Mobile apps can provide services in multiple languages
- Digital platforms can reduce transportation barriers

Anonymity and Reduced Stigma:

- Online services may feel less stigmatizing for some populations
- Anonymous screening can help identify needs without requiring disclosure
- Digital platforms may feel safer for discussing sensitive topics

Challenges and Limitations

Digital Divide:

- Limited access to technology in low-income communities
- Unreliable internet service in rural areas
- Lack of digital literacy skills
- Language barriers in predominantly English-language platforms

Cultural Appropriateness:

- Most mental health apps developed for majority populations
- Limited availability of culturally adapted digital interventions
- Concerns about data privacy and government surveillance
- Technology may not fit cultural preferences for in-person healing

Best Practices for Culturally Responsive Technology

- Ensure digital platforms are available in multiple languages
- Include diverse images and examples in apps and websites
- Test technology with community members before implementation
- Provide technical support and training for users

- Maintain options for in-person services alongside digital offerings

The Future of Culturally Responsive Care

The field of culturally responsive mental health care continues to evolve as research advances our understanding of how culture influences mental health and as demographics continue to shift.

Emerging Trends

Precision Medicine Approaches: Research is beginning to identify how genetic factors interact with cultural and environmental factors to influence mental health and treatment response.

Community-Defined Evidence: There's growing recognition that communities should define what constitutes evidence of effective interventions, not just researchers.

Decolonizing Mental Health: Movement to center indigenous and traditional healing practices rather than simply adapting Western interventions.

Intersectionality Focus: Increased attention to how multiple identities (race, gender, sexuality, class) interact to influence mental health experiences.

Ongoing Challenges

Despite progress, significant challenges remain:

- Limited funding for culturally adapted interventions
- Workforce diversity lags behind population changes
- Structural racism continues to create barriers to care
- Immigration policies create fear and reduce service utilization
- Mental health stigma persists in many communities

Your Role in Creating Change

As a pediatric mental health provider, you have opportunities to advance culturally responsive care:

Direct Practice:

- Provide culturally humble, affirming care to all families
- Continuously develop your cultural competency skills
- Advocate for individual children and families
- Build relationships with diverse communities

Professional Development:

- Seek additional training in cultural competency
- Participate in research on culturally adapted interventions
- Mentor other providers in cultural responsiveness
- Join professional organizations focused on health equity

Systems Change:

- Advocate for organizational policies that promote equity
- Participate in quality improvement efforts to reduce disparities
- Support hiring and retention of diverse staff
- Work with communities to design responsive services

Final Reflections

Cultural competency in pediatric mental health isn't just about learning facts about different ethnic groups or memorizing culturally appropriate greetings. It's about fundamentally shifting how we understand mental health challenges and recognizing that healing occurs within cultural contexts that give life meaning.

Every child and family brings a unique cultural perspective shaped by race, ethnicity, religion, sexual orientation, gender identity, socioeconomic status, and countless other factors. Our job isn't to become experts on every culture—that's impossible. Instead, we must become skilled at cultural humility: approaching each family with curiosity rather than assumptions, asking about their cultural background and preferences, and adapting our approaches to fit their worldview.

Remember Aaliyah, Alex, and Joaquín from the beginning of this chapter? Each of their stories illustrates how cultural factors influence mental health experiences and treatment engagement. Aaliyah's family's concerns about privacy reflect both cultural values and realistic fears about stigma in their community. Alex's hesitation about disclosure comes from valid concerns about safety and acceptance. Joaquín's testing of boundaries makes sense given his experiences with adults who've failed to keep their promises.

Culturally responsive care for these youth would look different in each case. Aaliyah might benefit from family-based interventions that honor her culture's collective approach to problem-solving. Alex needs LGBTQ+ affirming care that validates their identity while helping them navigate family relationships. Joaquín requires trauma-informed approaches that understand his behavior as adaptive responses to chronic instability.

The children and families we serve have survived tremendous challenges and demonstrated remarkable resilience. They possess cultural wisdom, healing traditions, and community connections that can support their recovery. Our role is to recognize these strengths, build upon them, and create space for healing to occur in culturally meaningful ways.

This work isn't easy. It requires ongoing self-examination, willingness to make mistakes and learn from them, and commitment to fighting systems that create and maintain disparities. But it's also deeply rewarding work that allows us to participate in healing that honors the full humanity and cultural richness of every child and family we serve.

Chapter 12: Family Systems and Parent Engagement

The family therapy session wasn't going as planned. Fourteen-year-old Emma sat with her arms crossed, glaring at her parents while they described her "out-of-control" behavior. Mom spoke rapidly about missed curfews and failing grades, while Dad sat silently, checking his phone. Emma's 10-year-old brother fidgeted in his chair, clearly wishing he were anywhere else.

"She never used to be like this," Mom insisted. "Ever since the divorce..." She trailed off, shooting a glance at her ex-husband. Dad finally looked up from his phone to mutter, "Maybe if you didn't undermine everything I try to do." Emma rolled her eyes. "Here we go again," she said under her breath.

The therapist took a deep breath, recognizing a familiar pattern. This family was stuck in cycles of blame and reactivity that kept everyone feeling frustrated and misunderstood. Emma's "problematic" behavior made perfect sense when viewed through a family systems lens—she was responding to the stress and conflict around her, perhaps even serving as a distraction from her parents' unresolved issues.

This scenario illustrates why pediatric mental health providers must understand family dynamics. Children don't exist in isolation—they're part of complex family systems where everyone influences everyone else. A child's symptoms often reflect family stress, communication patterns, or unmet needs that extend far beyond the identified patient.

Family Systems Theory

Family systems theory revolutionized how mental health professionals understand psychological problems. Instead of viewing issues as residing within individuals, systems theory recognizes that families operate as interconnected units where changes in one part affect the whole system.

Key Principles of Family Systems Theory

Wholeness: The family system is greater than the sum of its individual members. You can't understand one person without understanding their family context.

Circular Causality: Rather than linear cause-and-effect relationships, family problems involve circular patterns where everyone contributes to maintaining problems.

Homeostasis: Families develop patterns of interaction that maintain stability, even when those patterns are problematic.

Boundaries: Healthy families have clear boundaries between subsystems (parent subsystem, child subsystem) while maintaining emotional connection.

Hierarchy: Functional families have clear leadership structure with parents in charge of major decisions and discipline.

Family Structures and Patterns

Families organize themselves in predictable ways that either support or undermine healthy development:

Enmeshed Families: Boundaries are blurred, with family members overly involved in each other's lives. Children may feel responsible for parents' emotions or marriages.

Disengaged Families: Boundaries are too rigid, with family members emotionally disconnected from each other. Children may feel isolated and unsupported.

Triangulation: When two family members have conflict, they involve a third person (often a child) to reduce tension. This puts children in inappropriate roles and maintains parental conflict.

Scapegoating: One family member (often the child with mental health symptoms) becomes the focus of family problems, allowing other members to avoid addressing their own issues.

Consider the Martinez family: 16-year-old Sofia has been struggling with depression since her parents' relationship became increasingly conflictual. Rather than address their marriage problems directly, Mom confides in Sofia about Dad's drinking, while Dad complains to Sofia about Mom's spending. Sofia feels responsible for holding the family together and can't focus on typical teenage concerns like school and friendships.

Family Assessment Strategies

Comprehensive family assessment helps providers understand how family dynamics contribute to children's mental health challenges and identifies strengths to build upon.

Structural Assessment

Understanding family structure involves mapping relationships, boundaries, and power dynamics:

Family Composition: Who lives in the home? Who are the important people in this child's life? *Subsystem Boundaries:* Are parents united in their leadership? Do children have age-appropriate responsibilities? *Hierarchy:* Who makes decisions? Are children parentified or given inappropriate power? *Alliances:* Are there coalitions that exclude some family members or cross generational boundaries?

Communication Patterns

How families communicate reveals important information about their functioning:

Communication Style: Direct vs. indirect, open vs. closed, validating vs. invalidating *Conflict Resolution:* How does the family handle disagreements? Are conflicts avoided or escalated? *Emotional Expression:* Are feelings acknowledged and accepted? Is emotional expression safe? *Listening Skills:* Do family members really hear each other or just wait for their turn to talk?

Family Roles and Rules

Every family has spoken and unspoken rules that govern behavior:

Explicit Rules: Family rules that are clearly stated ("No phones during dinner") *Implicit Rules:* Unspoken expectations ("Don't talk about Dad's drinking") *Role Flexibility:* Can family members take on different roles as needed? *Role Clarity:* Does everyone understand their responsibilities and boundaries?

Genograms: Mapping Family Relationships

Genograms are visual representations of family structure and relationships across generations. They help identify patterns, strengths, and areas of concern that might not be obvious through conversation alone.

Basic Genogram Symbols:

Males: Represented by squares *Females:* Represented by circles *Unknown gender:* Represented by triangles *Marriages:* Connected by horizontal lines *Children:* Connected to parents by vertical lines *Divorces:* Shown by diagonal lines through marriage line *Deaths:* Indicated by X through the symbol

Relationship Lines:

173

Close relationships: Three parallel lines *Conflictual relationships:* Jagged lines *Cut-off relationships:* Lines with breaks *Enmeshed relationships:* Curved lines around symbols

Genograms can reveal patterns like:

- Multigenerational mental health challenges
- Relationship patterns that repeat across generations
- Family strengths and resources
- Cultural and ethnic influences
- Trauma and loss experiences

When creating genograms with families, therapists often discover important information that wasn't initially disclosed. A mother might realize that her son's anxiety symptoms began around the same time her father was diagnosed with cancer. A father might recognize that his harsh discipline style mirrors how he was raised by his own authoritarian father.

Evidence-Based Family Interventions

Research has identified several family-based interventions that effectively address children's mental health challenges by changing family dynamics and improving relationships.

Triple P: Positive Parenting Program

Triple P is a multilevel parenting program designed to prevent behavioral and emotional problems in children while promoting positive family relationships.

Triple P Principles:

- Ensuring a safe and engaging environment
- Creating a positive learning environment
- Using assertive discipline
- Having realistic expectations
- Taking care of yourself as a parent

Program Levels:

Level 1: Universal media-based parenting information *Level 2:* Brief primary care consultations for minor concerns *Level 3:* Narrow-focus parenting sessions for specific problems *Level 4:* Intensive individual or group parenting programs *Level 5:* Enhanced family intervention for families with multiple risk factors

Triple P has been evaluated in numerous studies and consistently shows improvements in:

- Children's behavioral and emotional problems
- Parent confidence and competence
- Family relationships and communication
- Parental stress and mental health

The program is particularly effective because it builds on parents' existing strengths while teaching specific skills for common challenges. Rather than telling parents what they're doing wrong, Triple P helps them discover more effective approaches.

The Incredible Years

The Incredible Years is a series of evidence-based programs designed to promote children's social and emotional competence and prevent conduct problems.

Program Components:

Parent Training: Teaches positive parenting strategies, effective discipline, and problem-solving skills *Child Training:* Builds children's social skills, emotional regulation, and problem-solving abilities *Teacher Training:* Helps educators create supportive classroom environments and manage behavioral challenges

Key Strategies:

- Child-directed play to strengthen relationships

- Praise and encouragement to build confidence
- Clear expectations and consistent consequences
- Problem-solving skills for handling conflicts
- Emotional coaching to help children understand feelings

Research demonstrates that Incredible Years programs reduce children's aggressive behavior, improve social skills, and strengthen parent-child relationships. The programs are particularly effective for families dealing with conduct problems, ADHD, and early behavioral challenges.

Multisystemic Therapy (MST)

MST is an intensive family-based intervention designed for adolescents with serious behavioral problems, including those at risk for out-of-home placement.

MST Principles:

- Problems are viewed within their systemic context
- Interventions target specific risk factors
- Treatment focuses on strengths and empowers families
- Interventions are present-focused and action-oriented
- Services are available 24/7 with small caseloads

Target Systems:

- Individual (adolescent psychological factors)
- Family (parenting practices, family structure)
- Peer (associations with deviant peers)
- School (academic performance, school engagement)
- Community (neighborhood factors, service coordination)

MST therapists work with families in their homes and communities, helping them develop skills to address problems across all relevant systems. The approach recognizes that adolescent behavioral problems rarely result from single causes and require comprehensive, coordinated responses.

Functional Family Therapy (FFT)

FFT is designed specifically for adolescents with behavioral problems and their families. The model focuses on changing family interaction patterns while building on existing family strengths.

Treatment Phases:

Engagement and Motivation: Building therapeutic relationships and increasing family motivation for change *Behavior Change:* Teaching specific skills and modifying problematic interaction patterns *Generalization:* Helping families apply new skills across different situations and maintain changes over time

Core Components:

- Reframing problems in relational terms rather than blaming individuals
- Building motivation by highlighting family strengths and possibilities
- Teaching communication and problem-solving skills
- Restructuring family relationships and boundaries
- Creating sustainable changes that prevent future problems

FFT has shown effectiveness in reducing adolescent behavioral problems, improving family relationships, and preventing future delinquency. The approach is particularly valuable because it helps families understand how their interaction patterns contribute to problems while providing concrete tools for change.

Parent-Child Interaction Therapy (PCIT)

PCIT is designed for families with young children (ages 2-7) who have behavioral problems. The intervention focuses on improving the quality of parent-child relationships and teaching parents effective behavior management skills.

Treatment Components:

177

Child-Directed Interaction (CDI): Parents learn to follow their child's lead in play, providing attention and praise for positive behaviors *Parent-Directed Interaction (PDI):* Parents learn to give effective commands and use consistent consequences

Unique Features:

- Therapist coaches parents through an earpiece while they interact with their child
- Parents must meet skill criteria before progressing to the next phase
- Treatment continues until parents demonstrate mastery of skills
- Live coaching provides immediate feedback and support

PCIT has strong research support for reducing child behavioral problems, improving parent-child relationships, and decreasing parental stress. The approach is particularly effective because parents practice new skills with their own children under expert guidance.

Parent Training and Support Strategies

Supporting parents is often the most effective way to help children with mental health challenges. Parents who feel confident and competent are better able to provide the consistent, nurturing care that promotes children's emotional wellbeing.

Core Parenting Skills

Positive Attention and Relationship Building

Strong parent-child relationships form the foundation for children's mental health. Key strategies include:

Special Time: Regular one-on-one time focused entirely on the child's interests *Active Listening:* Really hearing and understanding children's perspectives *Emotional Validation:* Acknowledging and accepting children's feelings *Physical Affection:* Appropriate hugs, cuddles, and physical closeness *Shared Activities:* Finding activities both parent and child enjoy

Consider Sarah, whose 8-year-old son Jake has been having behavioral problems at school. Through parent training, Sarah learned to spend 15 minutes daily in child-directed play with Jake. During this time, she follows his lead, avoids giving directions, and provides lots of positive attention. Within weeks, Jake's behavior improved both at home and school as their relationship strengthened.

Effective Communication Strategies

Reflective Listening: Repeating back what you hear to ensure understanding *"I" Statements:* Expressing your feelings without blaming ("I feel frustrated when..." rather than "You always...") *Problem-Solving Together:* Involving children in finding solutions to family challenges *Family Meetings:* Regular times for discussing concerns and making decisions together

Behavior Management Techniques

Clear Expectations: Rules and expectations that are specific, achievable, and consistently enforced *Natural and Logical Consequences:* Consequences that relate directly to the behavior and help children learn *Positive Reinforcement:* Catching children doing things right and acknowledging their efforts *Planned Ignoring:* Not responding to attention-seeking behaviors while continuing to attend to positive behaviors

Addressing Common Parenting Challenges

Sibling Rivalry and Competition

Sibling conflicts can create significant family stress and contribute to children's behavioral and emotional problems. Effective strategies include:

- Spending individual time with each child
- Avoiding comparisons between siblings
- Teaching conflict resolution skills
- Focusing on cooperation rather than competition
- Addressing underlying needs that drive sibling rivalry

Technology and Screen Time Issues

Modern parents face unique challenges managing children's technology use. Balanced approaches include:

- Creating family media agreements with clear expectations
- Modeling healthy technology use
- Providing engaging alternatives to screen time
- Using parental controls appropriately
- Addressing cyberbullying and online safety concerns

Discipline That Teaches Rather Than Punishes

Effective discipline focuses on teaching appropriate behavior rather than simply punishing mistakes:

Time-In Instead of Time-Out: Staying connected with children while helping them calm down *Natural Consequences:* Allowing children to experience the results of their choices *Problem-Solving Approach:* Working together to find solutions when problems occur *Restorative Justice:* Helping children make amends when they've hurt others

Working with Complex Family Situations

Many families face additional challenges that complicate mental health treatment and require specialized approaches.

Divorce and Separation

Parental divorce affects approximately 40% of children and can significantly impact their mental health and development. However, it's not divorce itself that harms children—it's the conflict, instability, and loss of support that often accompany divorce.

Risk Factors:

- High levels of parental conflict before, during, and after divorce
- Economic hardship following divorce
- Loss of contact with one parent
- Multiple transitions and changes
- Being caught in the middle of parental conflicts

Protective Factors:

- Low levels of ongoing conflict between parents
- Maintaining relationships with both parents when safe and appropriate
- Economic stability
- Consistent routines and expectations
- Age-appropriate explanations about the divorce

Supporting Children Through Divorce:

For Parents:

- Keep conflict away from children
- Reassure children that the divorce is not their fault
- Maintain routines and consistency as much as possible
- Allow children to express their feelings without judgment
- Avoid using children as messengers or confidants

For Providers:

- Help parents understand divorce's impact on children
- Teach co-parenting skills and communication strategies
- Address children's feelings of guilt, anger, and sadness
- Support family reorganization and adjustment
- Connect families with divorce support resources

Parental Mental Illness

When parents struggle with mental health challenges, children are at increased risk for developing their own mental health problems. However, many children of parents with mental illness develop resilience and coping skills that serve them well throughout life.

Impact on Children:

- Increased risk for anxiety, depression, and behavioral problems
- Role reversals where children take care of parents
- Inconsistent caregiving and emotional support
- Stigma and shame about family mental health challenges
- Academic and social difficulties

Supporting Families:

For Parents:

- Encourage treatment for parental mental health concerns
- Help parents develop age-appropriate explanations for children
- Teach parents to recognize when their symptoms affect their parenting
- Connect parents with peer support and resources
- Support parents in maintaining their parental role even during difficult times

For Children:

- Provide age-appropriate education about mental illness
- Help children understand that parents' illness is not their fault
- Teach coping skills for managing family stress
- Connect children with supportive adults outside the family
- Address any parentification or inappropriate responsibilities

Substance Use in Families

Parental substance use affects millions of children and significantly increases their risk for mental health, behavioral, and academic problems.

Impact on Children:

- Inconsistent and unpredictable caregiving
- Exposure to dangerous situations and people
- Economic instability and housing insecurity
- Trauma from witnessing violence or overdoses
- Increased risk for developing their own substance use problems

Family Recovery Approaches:

- Treat the whole family, not just the person with addiction
- Address trauma and mental health issues alongside substance use
- Build family communication and coping skills
- Connect families with recovery community supports
- Provide ongoing support during early recovery when relapse risk is highest

Blended Families and Step-Parenting

When parents remarry and form blended families, children must adjust to new family structures, relationships, and expectations.

Common Challenges:

- Loyalty conflicts between biological and step-parents
- Different rules and expectations between households
- Sibling relationships with step-siblings
- Loss of special relationship with single parent
- Adjustment to new family routines and traditions

Supporting Blended Family Success:

- Take time to build relationships before assuming parental authority
- Maintain children's relationships with both biological parents when appropriate
- Create new family traditions while honoring existing ones
- Establish clear roles and expectations for all family members
- Seek professional support during the adjustment period

Engaging Reluctant or Resistant Families

Not all families eagerly participate in mental health treatment. Many come to services involuntarily through school referrals, court orders, or child welfare involvement. Others may be willing but skeptical about therapy's effectiveness.

Understanding Resistance

Resistance often makes sense when viewed from families' perspectives:

Previous Negative Experiences: Families may have had unhelpful or harmful experiences with mental health services *Cultural Mistrust:* Some communities have valid reasons to mistrust helping systems *Shame and Stigma:* Mental health challenges can feel like personal failures or character flaws *Fear of Judgment:* Parents worry that providers will blame them for their children's problems *Practical Barriers:* Transportation, work schedules, and childcare can make attendance difficult

Engagement Strategies

Start Where the Family Is: Begin with problems families identify as important rather than provider concerns *Emphasize Strengths:* Highlight what families are doing well before addressing problems *Collaborate Rather Than Prescribe:* Work with families to develop solutions rather than telling them what to do *Address Practical Needs:* Help with concrete concerns like housing or food before focusing on therapy goals *Respect Cultural Values:* Understand how families' cultural backgrounds influence their help-seeking

Building Trust Over Time

Trust develops through consistent, reliable interactions where families feel heard, respected, and supported. Key strategies include:

- Following through on commitments, no matter how small
- Admitting when you don't know something rather than pretending expertise
- Advocating for families in other systems when appropriate
- Respecting families' expertise about their own situations
- Maintaining appropriate boundaries while showing genuine care

Consider the Johnson family, who came to therapy reluctantly after their 12-year-old daughter was suspended for fighting. Mom was defensive and angry, insisting that school officials were picking on her daughter because of her race. Rather than challenging this perception, the therapist listened carefully and acknowledged the reality of racial bias in schools. Only after Mom felt heard and understood was she willing to explore how to help her daughter succeed despite these challenges.

Supporting Diverse Family Structures

Families come in many different forms, and effective family therapy must adapt to various structures and compositions.

Single-Parent Families

Single parents face unique challenges including:

- Financial stress and limited resources
- Lack of parenting support and backup
- Social isolation and limited adult interaction
- Balancing work and parenting responsibilities

- Managing their own stress while supporting children

Support strategies include:

- Connecting single parents with peer support groups
- Building extended support networks of family and friends
- Teaching stress management and self-care skills
- Advocating for workplace flexibility and family-friendly policies
- Addressing any guilt or self-blame about family structure

Grandparents as Primary Caregivers

Increasingly, grandparents are raising grandchildren due to parental death, incarceration, addiction, or inability to care for children.

Unique challenges include:

- Physical health limitations and aging concerns
- Financial strain on fixed incomes
- Legal complications regarding custody and decision-making
- Grief and loss related to their adult child's problems
- Generation gap in understanding current child-rearing practices

Support approaches include:

- Connecting grandparents with kinship care support groups
- Providing education about current child development and mental health understanding
- Addressing legal and custody issues
- Supporting grandparents' own health and wellbeing
- Helping grandchildren process their complex family situation

LGBTQ+ Parents and Families

LGBTQ+ families face unique stressors related to discrimination, legal challenges, and lack of social support.

Considerations include:

- Legal protections for non-biological parents
- Discrimination in schools and healthcare settings
- Limited representation in children's books and media
- Explaining family structure to others
- Managing coming-out processes if parents are not open about their identity

Affirming support includes:

- Using inclusive language that reflects family structure
- Understanding legal vulnerabilities LGBTQ+ families face
- Connecting families with LGBTQ+ affirming resources and support groups
- Advocating for families in discriminatory situations
- Celebrating the strengths and resilience of LGBTQ+ families

Family Communication and Problem-Solving Skills

Teaching families effective communication and problem-solving skills provides tools they can use long after therapy ends.

Communication Skills Training

Active Listening Techniques: *Paraphrasing:* "What I hear you saying is..." *Reflecting Feelings:* "It sounds like you're feeling..." *Asking Clarifying Questions:* "Can you help me understand..." *Summarizing:* "So the main points seem to be..."

Expressing Feelings and Needs: *"I" Statements:* "I feel... when... because... I need..." *Specific Rather Than General:* "When you leave dishes in the sink" rather than "You're always messy" *Timing:* Choosing appropriate times for difficult conversations *Tone and Body Language:* Matching nonverbal communication with words

Managing Conflict Constructively: *Ground Rules:* No name-calling, interrupting, or bringing up past grievances *Taking Breaks:* Stepping away when emotions get too heated *Finding Common Ground:* Identifying shared goals and values *Compromise and Negotiation:* Finding solutions that meet everyone's needs

Family Problem-Solving Process

Step 1: Define the Problem

- What exactly is the problem?
- Who is affected and how?
- When does the problem occur?
- What makes it better or worse?

Step 2: Brainstorm Solutions

- Generate as many ideas as possible without judging
- Encourage creative and unusual solutions
- Build on each other's ideas
- Write down all suggestions

Step 3: Evaluate Options

- What are the pros and cons of each solution?
- Which solutions are realistic and feasible?
- What resources would each solution require?
- Which solutions align with family values?

Step 4: Choose and Implement

- Select the solution that seems most promising
- Make a specific plan for implementation
- Identify potential obstacles and how to address them
- Set a timeline for trying the solution

Step 5: Evaluate and Adjust

- How well is the solution working?
- What modifications are needed?
- Should you try a different approach?
- What have you learned for future problems?

This structured approach helps families move beyond arguing about problems to actively working together on solutions.

Crisis Management in Family Systems

When families face crises, their usual coping strategies may become overwhelmed, requiring additional support and intervention.

Types of Family Crises

Developmental Crises:

- Normal life transitions that create stress (births, adolescence, launching young adults)
- Require adaptation to new roles and relationships
- Often resolved with time and support

Situational Crises:

- Unexpected events that disrupt family functioning (job loss, illness, accidents)
- Require immediate problem-solving and resource mobilization
- May result in positive growth or lasting difficulties

Chronic Stressors:

- Ongoing challenges that wear down family resources (poverty, illness, disability)
- Require long-term coping strategies and support
- May lead to family burnout and breakdown without intervention

Crisis Intervention Principles

Immediate Safety: Ensure all family members are physically and emotionally safe *Stabilization:* Help families regain a sense of control and predictability *Resource Mobilization:* Connect families with practical and emotional supports *Meaning-Making:* Help families understand and process the crisis experience *Future Planning:* Develop strategies for preventing or managing future crises

Building Family Resilience

Resilient families bounce back from adversity and often emerge stronger than before. Key characteristics include:

- Flexibility and adaptability in facing challenges
- Open communication and problem-solving skills
- Strong emotional bonds and mutual support
- Sense of shared meaning and purpose
- Connection to external supports and resources
- Optimism and hope for the future

Providers can help families build resilience by:

- Identifying and strengthening existing family resources
- Teaching coping and problem-solving skills
- Connecting families with community supports
- Helping families find meaning in their challenges
- Celebrating family strengths and achievements

Technology and Modern Family Life

Digital technology has fundamentally changed family life, creating new opportunities for connection while also introducing new challenges and stressors.

Benefits of Technology for Families

- Staying connected with extended family across distances
- Access to educational resources and online learning
- Entertainment and shared activities
- Support groups and communities for families facing challenges
- Tools for organization and family coordination

Technology-Related Family Challenges

Screen Time Battles:

- Disagreements about appropriate amounts and types of screen time
- Difficulty balancing online and offline activities
- Competition between family time and device time

Cyberbullying and Online Safety:

- Protecting children from online predators and inappropriate content
- Addressing cyberbullying and digital drama
- Teaching digital citizenship and responsible online behavior

Social Media and Identity:

- Pressure to present perfect family images online
- Comparison with other families on social media
- Impact of social media on children's self-esteem and body image

Creating Healthy Technology Boundaries

Family Media Agreements: Collaborative rules about when, where, and how technology is used *Tech-Free Zones and Times:* Designated spaces and times without devices (dinner table, bedrooms) *Modeling Healthy Use:* Parents demonstrating balanced technology habits *Regular Family Conversations:* Ongoing discussions about digital experiences and challenges

Working with Schools and Other Systems

Children's mental health challenges often affect their performance in school, making collaboration with educational systems essential.

Common School-Related Mental Health Issues

- Academic underachievement despite adequate ability
- Behavioral problems that interfere with learning
- Social difficulties and peer relationship challenges
- School avoidance and anxiety about academic performance
- Attention and concentration difficulties

Collaboration Strategies

Information Sharing: Working with families to share relevant information with schools (with appropriate consents) *Treatment Planning:* Including educational goals in mental health treatment plans *Consultation:* Providing guidance to teachers about managing mental health challenges in classroom settings *Advocacy:* Supporting families in obtaining appropriate educational services and accommodations

Special Education and 504 Plans

Some children with mental health challenges qualify for special education services or accommodations under Section 504:

Individualized Education Program (IEP): For children whose mental health challenges significantly impact educational performance *504 Plan:* For children who need accommodations to access education but don't qualify for special education *Common Accommodations:* Extended time on tests, breaks during instruction, modified assignments, counseling services

Measuring Family Progress and Outcomes

Effective family therapy includes ongoing assessment of progress toward treatment goals.

Family Functioning Measures

Family Assessment Device (FAD): Evaluates family functioning across multiple dimensions *Family Environment Scale (FES):* Assesses social environment characteristics of families *Parenting Stress Index:* Measures stress in parent-child relationships *Family Adaptability and Cohesion Evaluation Scales (FACES):* Assesses family cohesion and flexibility

Goal Setting and Progress Monitoring

SMART Goals: Specific, Measurable, Achievable, Relevant, Time-bound objectives *Scaling Questions:* Rating progress on a scale of 1-10 to track changes over time *Behavioral Observations:* Tracking specific behaviors and interactions *Family Feedback:* Regular check-ins about what's working and what needs adjustment

Celebrating Success and Maintaining Changes

- Acknowledging progress and celebrating achievements
- Identifying what strategies were most helpful
- Planning for setbacks and challenges
- Developing long-term maintenance strategies
- Connecting families with ongoing support resources

Fostering Hope and Healing in Families

Family therapy is ultimately about helping families rediscover their capacity for love, support, and connection. Even families facing significant challenges possess strengths and resources that can be mobilized for healing.

Strength-Based Approaches

Rather than focusing solely on problems and deficits, effective family therapy identifies and builds upon existing family strengths:

- Natural resilience and coping abilities
- Cultural wisdom and traditions
- Extended family and community connections
- Previous experiences overcoming adversity
- Individual talents and abilities of family members

Creating New Narratives

Families often become stuck in problem-saturated stories about themselves. Family therapy helps create new narratives that emphasize:

- Growth and change rather than fixed characteristics
- Collaborative efforts rather than individual blame
- Hope for the future rather than despair about the past
- Unique outcomes that contradict problem stories
- Preferred identities and relationships

The Ripple Effect of Family Healing

When families heal, the benefits extend far beyond the immediate family system:

- Children develop healthier templates for their own future relationships
- Extended family relationships often improve
- Community connections and support networks strengthen
- Cycles of trauma and dysfunction can be interrupted across generations
- Families become resources for other families facing similar challenges

My Thoughts on Family-Centered Care

Remember Emma and her family from the beginning of this chapter? Through family therapy, they began to understand how their divorce process had created impossible positions for both children. Emma's "acting out" wasn't just typical teenage rebellion—it was her way of expressing pain about her family's changes and trying to get her parents' attention back on parenting rather than their conflicts.

As the parents learned to communicate about co-parenting without attacking each other, Emma no longer felt responsible for protecting either parent. Her brother stopped feeling invisible and began getting the attention he needed. Most importantly, both children learned that their parents' problems weren't their fault and that they could count on both parents to continue loving and supporting them despite the divorce.

This transformation didn't happen overnight. It required patience, skill, and commitment from everyone involved. But the changes were lasting because they addressed the underlying family dynamics that had been maintaining everyone's distress.

Family-centered care recognizes that children's mental health cannot be separated from their family relationships and experiences. When we help families develop stronger connections, better communication, and more effective problem-solving skills, we create environments where children naturally thrive.

The families we serve bring tremendous wisdom, strength, and love to the therapeutic process. Our job is to help them rediscover these resources and use them to create the kinds of relationships and family life they truly want. When we get this right, we don't just treat symptoms—we help families become sources of healing and growth for all their members.

Chapter 13: Practice Settings Across the Continuum

The phone rang at 2:47 AM in the pediatric emergency department. "We have a 15-year-old coming in by ambulance," the paramedic reported. "Parents found him after an overdose attempt. He's conscious but pretty upset."

Twenty minutes later, Jake arrived with his terrified parents trailing behind the stretcher. The emergency psychiatry nurse began her assessment while the medical team stabilized his condition. This was Jake's entry point into what would become a journey through multiple levels of mental healthcare—from emergency services to inpatient treatment, then transitioning to intensive outpatient care, and eventually connecting with school-based mental health services.

Jake's story illustrates something important about pediatric mental health: care happens across a continuum of settings, each designed to meet different levels of need and intensity. Understanding these various practice environments isn't just academic knowledge—it's essential for providing coordinated, effective care that meets children and families where they are.

The Continuum of Care Model

Mental health services exist on a continuum from least restrictive to most intensive interventions. This continuum ensures that children receive appropriate care that matches their current needs while preserving their connections to family, school, and community whenever possible.

Levels of Care Intensity

The continuum typically includes these levels, from least to most restrictive:

- Prevention and early intervention programs
- Outpatient therapy (individual, family, group)
- Intensive outpatient programs (IOP)
- Partial hospitalization programs (PHP)
- Residential treatment
- Inpatient hospitalization
- Emergency and crisis services

Each level serves different purposes and populations. A child might move between levels as their needs change, or receive services from multiple levels simultaneously.

Key Principles Guiding Level of Care Decisions

Least Restrictive Environment: Children should receive care in the setting that meets their needs while allowing maximum freedom and community connection.

Medical Necessity: The level of care must be justified by the child's clinical condition and functional impairment.

Family Involvement: Whenever possible, treatment should strengthen rather than replace family relationships.

Cultural Responsiveness: Services should match families' cultural values and preferences.

Developmental Appropriateness: Treatment approaches must fit the child's cognitive, emotional, and social development.

Inpatient Psychiatric Units

Inpatient units provide the most intensive level of mental health care, typically reserved for children who pose immediate danger to themselves or others, or who are so impaired they can't function safely in less restrictive settings.

Who Gets Admitted

Inpatient admission criteria generally include:

- Active suicidal or homicidal ideation with plan and means
- Psychosis or severe disorganization affecting safety
- Severe mood episodes with significant functional impairment
- Eating disorder with medical complications
- Inability to care for basic needs due to mental illness
- Failure to respond to less intensive interventions

The Inpatient Environment

Pediatric psychiatric units differ significantly from adult units, with environments specifically designed for developing minds and bodies.

Physical Environment:

- Age-appropriate decorations and furniture
- Spaces for both individual and group activities
- Educational areas for continuing schoolwork
- Family meeting rooms
- Sensory regulation spaces

Daily Structure: Most inpatient units follow predictable schedules that provide safety and stability:

- Morning community meetings
- Individual therapy sessions
- Group therapy (multiple types)
- Educational services
- Recreational therapy
- Family therapy sessions

- Medication management
- Evening wrap-up activities

Length of Stay: Average inpatient stays have decreased dramatically over the past decades, now typically lasting 5-10 days. This short timeframe focuses on:

- Crisis stabilization
- Safety planning
- Medication adjustments
- Discharge planning to appropriate community services

Multidisciplinary Team Approach

Inpatient care involves multiple specialists working together:

Psychiatrists: Medical doctors who diagnose mental health conditions and prescribe medications *Psychiatric Nurses:* Provide direct care, medication administration, and therapeutic relationships *Social Workers:* Assess family dynamics, coordinate discharge planning, and connect families with community resources *Psychologists:* Conduct psychological testing and provide specialized therapy *Recreational Therapists:* Use activities and play to promote healing and skill development *Educational Staff:* Ensure children don't fall behind academically during hospitalization *Milieu Staff:* Trained in therapeutic communication and behavior management

Challenges in Inpatient Care

Despite its necessity for some children, inpatient care faces several challenges:

Limited Bed Availability: Many communities have insufficient pediatric psychiatric beds, leading to long emergency department stays.

Insurance Restrictions: Pressure to discharge quickly may not allow adequate stabilization.

Family Disruption: Separation from family can be traumatic, especially for younger children.

Stigma: Psychiatric hospitalization still carries significant stigma in many communities.

Continuity of Care: Connecting inpatient treatment with ongoing community services can be difficult.

Consider Maria, a 13-year-old admitted after a serious suicide attempt. During her seven-day stay, the team focused on safety, medication adjustment for her depression, and family therapy to address communication patterns. The social worker spent considerable time coordinating with her outpatient therapist and school to ensure smooth transition back to her community supports.

Outpatient and Community-Based Services

Most children with mental health challenges receive care in outpatient settings, which allow them to remain with their families and continue school while receiving treatment.

Types of Outpatient Services

Individual Therapy: One-on-one sessions between therapist and child, typically lasting 45-60 minutes. Common approaches include:

- Cognitive Behavioral Therapy (CBT)
- Play therapy for younger children
- Dialectical Behavior Therapy (DBT) for adolescents
- Trauma-focused therapies

Family Therapy: Sessions involving multiple family members to address relationship dynamics and communication patterns.

Group Therapy: Children with similar challenges meet together with a therapist to share experiences and learn skills. Common groups include:

- Social skills training
- Anger management
- Grief and loss support
- Substance abuse treatment

Medication Management: Regular appointments with psychiatrists or psychiatric nurse practitioners to prescribe, monitor, and adjust psychiatric medications.

Community Mental Health Centers

Community Mental Health Centers (CMHCs) serve as the backbone of public mental health services, providing care regardless of families' ability to pay.

Services Typically Offered:

- Individual and family therapy
- Group therapy programs
- Psychiatric services
- Case management
- Crisis intervention
- Peer support services

Populations Served: CMHCs often serve families who face multiple challenges including poverty, lack of insurance, transportation barriers, and complex mental health needs.

Challenges:

- High caseloads limiting session frequency
- Staff turnover affecting continuity
- Limited resources for specialized services
- Long waiting lists for initial appointments

Private Practice Settings

Many children receive mental health services through private practitioners, including psychologists, licensed clinical social workers, marriage and family therapists, and psychiatrists.

Advantages:

- Often shorter wait times for appointments
- More flexibility in treatment approaches
- Greater continuity with same provider
- Comfortable office environments

Limitations:

- Cost barriers for uninsured families
- Limited availability in rural areas
- May have less experience with severe mental illness
- Fewer wraparound services available

Intensive Outpatient and Partial Hospitalization Programs

Between traditional outpatient care and inpatient hospitalization exist intermediate levels of care that provide intensive services while allowing children to remain at home.

Intensive Outpatient Programs (IOPs)

IOPs typically involve 9-12 hours of treatment per week, usually spread across 3-4 days. Services commonly include:

- Individual therapy sessions
- Group therapy (multiple types)
- Family therapy
- Psychiatric services
- Skills training groups

Typical Schedule: Many IOPs run after school hours (4:00-7:00 PM) or on weekends to minimize disruption to education.

Target Population:

- Children stepping down from higher levels of care
- Those who need more support than weekly outpatient therapy
- Families in crisis who want to avoid hospitalization

Partial Hospitalization Programs (PHPs)

PHPs provide hospital-level care during daytime hours (typically 6-8 hours per day, 5 days per week) while allowing children to sleep at home.

Services Include:

- Daily individual therapy
- Multiple group therapy sessions
- Psychiatric services with frequent medication monitoring
- Educational services
- Family therapy and education
- Crisis planning and safety skills

Benefits:

- Intensive treatment without family separation
- Continued connection to community supports
- Less stigma than inpatient hospitalization
- Often less expensive than inpatient care

Consider Alex, a 16-year-old with severe depression who wasn't sleeping, eating poorly, and having passive suicidal thoughts. Rather than inpatient admission, Alex enrolled in a PHP where they received daily therapy, medication adjustments, and family support while sleeping at home each night. After three weeks, Alex transitioned to an IOP and then to weekly outpatient therapy.

School-Based Mental Health Services

Schools have become central to identifying and addressing children's mental health needs, given that children spend most of their waking hours in educational settings.

Models of School-Based Mental Health

Traditional School Counseling: School counselors provide brief counseling, crisis intervention, and referrals to community services. However, they often have large caseloads and multiple non-counseling duties.

School-Based Health Centers: Comprehensive health clinics located on school campuses that often include mental health services alongside medical care.

Embedded Mental Health Clinicians: Community mental health organizations place therapists and other clinicians directly in schools to provide services.

Consultation Models: Mental health professionals consult with school staff about specific students and provide training on mental health topics.

Advantages of School-Based Services

Accessibility: Services are available where children already spend their time, eliminating transportation barriers.

Early Identification: School staff can identify mental health concerns early and connect children with services quickly.

Reduced Stigma: Receiving services at school may feel more normalized and less stigmatizing.

Academic Integration: Mental health providers can work directly with teachers to support academic success.

Family Engagement: Schools may have better relationships with some families than traditional mental health settings.

Common School-Based Interventions

Individual Counseling: Brief therapy sessions addressing specific concerns like anxiety, depression, or behavioral problems.

Group Interventions:

- Social skills training
- Anger management
- Grief and loss support
- Substance abuse prevention

Crisis Intervention: Immediate response to mental health crises occurring during school hours.

Consultation: Working with teachers and administrators to develop strategies for supporting students with mental health challenges.

Prevention Programs: Universal interventions addressing topics like bullying prevention, emotional regulation, and stress management.

Challenges in School-Based Mental Health

Confidentiality Issues: Balancing student privacy with school safety requirements and parent involvement.

Role Confusion: Clarifying the relationship between mental health services and educational goals.

Sustainability: Securing ongoing funding for mental health programs in schools with competing budget priorities.

Staff Training: Ensuring school personnel understand mental health issues and appropriate referral processes.

Think about Sarah, a 10-year-old who started having panic attacks at school after her parents' divorce. The embedded therapist was able to see Sarah twice weekly during lunch periods, teach her coping skills for managing anxiety, and work with her teacher to create a signal system for when Sarah needed breaks. This immediate, accessible support prevented Sarah's anxiety from escalating to the point of school avoidance.

Integrated Care Models

The recognition that physical and mental health are interconnected has led to various integrated care models that address both types of needs simultaneously.

Primary Care Integration

Many children with mental health concerns are first seen in pediatric primary care settings. Integrated models place mental health professionals directly in medical offices or create strong collaboration between medical and mental health providers.

Co-located Services: Mental health clinicians work in the same physical space as medical providers, allowing for immediate consultation and referral.

Behavioral Health Consultants: Brief consultation services where mental health professionals provide assessment and recommendations during medical visits.

Collaborative Care Models: Structured approaches where primary care providers, mental health specialists, and care managers work together to treat mental health conditions.

Benefits of Integration

Reduced Stigma: Families may be more comfortable accessing mental health services in medical settings.

Early Identification: Medical providers can screen for mental health concerns during routine visits.

Coordinated Treatment: Physical and mental health conditions can be addressed simultaneously.

Improved Access: Families already have relationships with medical providers and may find it easier to access integrated services.

Challenges of Integration

Training Needs: Medical providers need training in mental health screening and basic interventions.

Documentation and Billing: Different requirements for mental health and medical services can create administrative burdens.

Space and Staffing: Adding mental health services requires additional resources and space.

Communication: Ensuring effective communication between different types of providers.

Telehealth and Digital Mental Health Services

Technology has transformed how mental health services are delivered, particularly accelerated by the COVID-19 pandemic.

Telepsychiatry and Teletherapy

Video-based therapy sessions allow mental health providers to connect with children and families regardless of geographic location.

Advantages:

- Increased access, especially in rural or underserved areas
- Reduced travel time and transportation barriers

- Ability to see children in their natural environments
- Continuity of care during illness or other disruptions
- Access to specialists not available locally

Challenges:

- Technology requirements and digital literacy needs
- Privacy and confidentiality concerns
- Difficulty building therapeutic relationships through screens
- Limited ability to assess nonverbal cues
- Insurance coverage variations

Best Practices for Telehealth with Children

Environmental Considerations:

- Ensuring private, quiet spaces for sessions
- Good lighting and camera positioning
- Reliable internet connections
- Backup communication plans

Engagement Strategies:

- Using interactive activities and games
- Involving parents appropriately based on child's age
- Shorter session lengths for younger children
- Creative use of technology features (screen sharing, virtual backgrounds)

Safety Protocols:

- Clear procedures for handling crises during telehealth sessions
- Knowledge of local emergency resources near client's location
- Documented safety plans accessible during sessions

Digital Mental Health Tools

Smartphone apps, online platforms, and digital therapeutic tools are increasingly used to supplement traditional mental health services.

Types of Digital Tools:

- Mood tracking and monitoring apps
- Meditation and mindfulness programs
- Cognitive behavioral therapy apps
- Crisis text lines and support chat services
- Educational resources about mental health

Benefits:

- 24/7 availability and accessibility
- Engaging formats that appeal to tech-savvy youth
- Lower cost than traditional therapy
- Anonymous options for stigma reduction
- Data collection for monitoring progress

Limitations:

- Limited research on effectiveness
- Privacy and data security concerns
- Lack of human connection
- Inappropriate for severe mental illness
- Digital divide affecting access

Consider Jake from our opening example. After his inpatient stay, Jake participated in an intensive outpatient program three evenings per week. He also used a mood tracking app to monitor his depression symptoms and connected with a crisis text line when he had suicidal thoughts between sessions. His therapist incorporated data from his app into their weekly sessions, and Jake found the 24/7 availability of the text line reassuring.

Quality Indicators Across Settings

Measuring quality in pediatric mental health services helps ensure children receive effective, appropriate care regardless of setting.

Structure Measures

These assess whether the right resources and systems are in place:

Staffing:

- Appropriate staff-to-patient ratios
- Staff credentials and training levels
- Availability of specialized services
- Cultural and linguistic competency of staff

Physical Environment:

- Safety features appropriate for children
- Age-appropriate spaces and materials
- Privacy protections
- Technology infrastructure

Policies and Procedures:

- Evidence-based treatment protocols
- Crisis intervention procedures
- Family involvement policies
- Cultural competency standards

Process Measures

These examine what happens during care delivery:

Access and Engagement:

- Time from referral to first appointment
- Show rates and engagement levels

- Cultural responsiveness of services
- Family satisfaction with communication

Clinical Care:

- Use of evidence-based treatments
- Appropriate assessment and screening
- Medication management protocols
- Discharge planning quality

Outcome Measures

These assess the results of mental health services:

Clinical Outcomes:

- Symptom reduction using standardized scales
- Functional improvement in home, school, and social settings
- Achievement of treatment goals
- Medication adherence and effectiveness

Service Utilization:

- Readmission rates
- Emergency service usage
- Treatment completion rates
- Transition success between levels of care

Experience Measures

These capture patients' and families' perspectives on care:

Patient and Family Satisfaction:

- Feeling heard and respected
- Cultural sensitivity of services
- Involvement in treatment planning
- Communication quality with providers

Provider Satisfaction:

- Job satisfaction and burnout rates
- Perceived effectiveness of treatments
- Adequacy of resources and support
- Professional development opportunities

Team Roles and Interdisciplinary Collaboration

Effective pediatric mental health care requires collaboration among professionals from multiple disciplines, each bringing unique expertise and perspectives.

Core Team Members

Psychiatrists and Psychiatric Nurse Practitioners:

- Diagnose mental health conditions
- Prescribe and monitor medications
- Provide medical oversight of treatment
- Assess for medical causes of psychiatric symptoms

Psychologists:

- Conduct psychological testing and assessment
- Provide individual, family, and group therapy
- Develop and implement behavioral interventions
- Consult on complex diagnostic questions

Licensed Clinical Social Workers:

- Provide individual, family, and group therapy
- Assess family and social systems
- Connect families with community resources
- Advocate for clients within various systems

Licensed Professional Counselors/Marriage and Family Therapists:

- Provide individual, family, and group therapy
- Specialize in specific therapeutic approaches
- Address relationship and communication issues
- Support families through transitions and crises

Psychiatric Nurses:

- Provide direct nursing care
- Administer and monitor medications
- Conduct therapeutic relationships
- Educate patients and families about mental health

Specialized Team Members

Case Managers:

- Coordinate services across multiple providers and systems
- Help families access resources and benefits
- Monitor treatment progress and outcomes
- Advocate for appropriate services

Peer Support Specialists:

- Individuals with lived experience providing support and mentorship
- Help reduce stigma and increase hope
- Model recovery and resilience
- Bridge gaps between professional services and community

Educational Staff:

- Ensure academic needs are met during treatment
- Coordinate with schools for smooth transitions
- Provide tutoring and educational support
- Address learning difficulties that may contribute to mental health challenges

Recreational and Expressive Therapists:

213

- Use art, music, dance, or recreational activities therapeutically
- Help children express emotions and develop skills
- Provide alternative communication methods for children who struggle with traditional talk therapy
- Build confidence and self-esteem through creative achievement

Effective Team Functioning

Clear Communication:

- Regular team meetings and case conferences
- Shared documentation systems
- Clear protocols for information sharing
- Defined roles and responsibilities

Collaborative Decision-Making:

- Shared treatment planning involving all disciplines
- Consensus building around major decisions
- Conflict resolution processes
- Family and patient involvement in team discussions

Quality Improvement:

- Regular review of outcomes and processes
- Team training and professional development
- System improvements based on data and feedback
- Peer review and consultation processes

Transitions and Continuity of Care

One of the biggest challenges in pediatric mental health is ensuring smooth transitions between different levels and settings of care.

Common Transition Points

Hospital to Community: Discharge from inpatient or emergency settings back to community-based care requires careful planning and coordination.

Between Levels of Care: Moving from intensive services to less restrictive settings, or stepping up to more intensive care when needed.

Age-Related Transitions: Transitioning from child to adolescent services, or from pediatric to adult mental health systems.

System Transitions: Moving between different service systems such as child welfare, juvenile justice, or educational settings.

Elements of Successful Transitions

Comprehensive Planning:

- Assessment of ongoing needs and risks
- Identification of appropriate next level of care
- Development of specific transition goals
- Timeline for transition activities

Communication and Coordination:

- Clear communication between sending and receiving providers
- Transfer of relevant clinical information
- Joint sessions or meetings when possible
- Warm handoffs between providers

Family Preparation and Support:

- Education about what to expect in new setting
- Addressing concerns and anxieties about change
- Involvement in transition planning
- Connection to peer support if available

Follow-up and Monitoring:

- Early contact after transition to assess adjustment
- Monitoring of symptoms and functioning
- Adjustment of treatment plans as needed
- Quick response to problems or concerns

Think about Emma, who transitioned from a residential treatment program back to her home community. Her transition plan included gradual home visits while still in residence, coordination between residential staff and her new outpatient therapist, enrollment in an intensive outpatient program for additional support, and weekly check-ins during the first month home. This careful planning helped Emma successfully maintain the progress she'd made in residential treatment.

Rural and Underserved Communities

Mental health services for children in rural and underserved communities face unique challenges that require creative solutions and adapted service delivery models.

Challenges in Rural Areas

Provider Shortages:

- Few mental health professionals available
- Limited specialized services for children
- High staff turnover rates
- Difficulty recruiting new providers

Geographic Barriers:

- Long distances to services
- Limited transportation options
- Weather-related access issues
- Time away from work or school for appointments

Cultural Factors:

- Stigma around mental health treatment
- Preference for informal support systems
- Religious or cultural beliefs about mental illness
- Close-knit communities where confidentiality is challenging

Innovative Service Delivery Models

Mobile Mental Health Services: Bringing services directly to communities through mobile clinics or traveling providers.

Telehealth and Technology: Using video conferencing and digital tools to connect rural children with specialists in urban areas.

School-Based Programs: Placing mental health services in schools where children already spend time and where stigma may be reduced.

Community Partnerships: Working with churches, community centers, and other trusted local organizations to provide services.

Training Local Providers: Building capacity by training primary care providers, teachers, and community members in mental health skills.

Emergency and Crisis Services

Mental health emergencies require immediate, specialized responses that can mean the difference between life and death for some children.

Types of Mental Health Crises

Suicidal Ideation or Attempts:

- Active thoughts of self-harm with plan or means
- Suicide attempts requiring medical attention

- Significant changes in suicide risk level

Homicidal Threats:

- Threats to harm others
- Access to weapons combined with violent thoughts
- History of violence with escalating behavior

Psychosis or Severe Disorganization:

- Loss of contact with reality
- Hallucinations or delusions affecting behavior
- Severe confusion or disorientation

Severe Substance Intoxication or Withdrawal:

- Overdoses requiring medical attention
- Withdrawal symptoms affecting safety
- Substance use combined with other risk factors

Crisis Response Systems

24/7 Crisis Hotlines: Telephone and text-based services providing immediate support and risk assessment.

Mobile Crisis Teams: Specially trained teams that can respond to mental health emergencies in community settings.

Emergency Department Services: Medical emergency departments equipped to handle psychiatric emergencies with specialized staff and protocols.

Crisis Stabilization Units: Short-term residential programs providing intensive support during mental health crises.

Best Practices in Crisis Response

Rapid Response:

- Quick access to crisis services
- Shortened wait times in emergency departments
- Immediate safety assessment and stabilization

De-escalation Techniques:

- Calm, non-threatening communication
- Validation of feelings and experiences
- Focus on immediate safety and support

Family Involvement:

- Including families in crisis planning when appropriate
- Providing support and education to family members
- Addressing family concerns and questions

Follow-up Planning:

- Connecting crisis services with ongoing treatment
- Safety planning for return to community
- Scheduled follow-up within 24-48 hours

Cultural Considerations Across Settings

Mental health services must be responsive to the diverse cultural backgrounds of children and families served.

Culturally Responsive Service Delivery

Staff Diversity: Hiring staff who reflect the cultural and linguistic diversity of the community served.

Language Access: Providing services in families' preferred languages through bilingual staff or professional interpreters.

Cultural Adaptation of Treatments: Modifying evidence-based treatments to fit cultural values and practices.

Community Engagement: Building relationships with cultural and community leaders to increase trust and access.

Flexible Service Delivery: Adapting service schedules, locations, and formats to fit cultural preferences and practical needs.

Addressing Cultural Barriers

Stigma Reduction:

- Community education about mental health
- Use of trusted community messengers
- Integration with other health and social services
- Focus on strengths and resilience

Trust Building:

- Consistent, reliable service delivery
- Transparency about treatment options and processes
- Respect for cultural values and practices
- Advocacy for families within other systems

Building a Better System of Care

Creating effective pediatric mental health services requires coordination and collaboration across all levels and settings of care.

System of Care Principles

Child and Family Centered: Services should be designed around the needs and preferences of children and families, not provider or system convenience.

Community Based: Services should be provided in or close to children's home communities whenever possible.

Culturally Competent: All services should be responsive to the cultural background and values of families served.

Individualized: Services should be tailored to each child's unique strengths, needs, and circumstances.

Least Restrictive: Children should receive care in the least restrictive setting that can safely and effectively meet their needs.

Keys to System Success

Strong Leadership: Committed leaders who can facilitate collaboration and drive system improvements.

Shared Vision: Common understanding of goals and values across all system participants.

Data-Driven Decision Making: Using outcome and performance data to guide service improvements and resource allocation.

Continuous Learning: Ongoing training, technical assistance, and quality improvement efforts.

Sustainable Financing: Stable funding mechanisms that support comprehensive services across the continuum.

Family and Youth Voice: Meaningful involvement of families and young people in system planning and evaluation.

Looking to the Future

The field of pediatric mental health continues to evolve, with new service delivery models, technologies, and approaches emerging regularly.

Emerging Trends

Prevention and Early Intervention: Increased focus on preventing mental health problems before they require intensive treatment.

Precision Medicine: Using genetic and other biological markers to tailor treatments to individual children.

Technology Integration: Continued expansion of telehealth, digital therapeutics, and AI-assisted assessment and treatment.

Trauma-Informed Care: System-wide adoption of approaches that recognize and respond to the impact of trauma.

Peer and Family Support: Expanded use of people with lived experience to provide support and advocacy.

Jake's journey through the mental health system took him from emergency services through inpatient care, intensive outpatient treatment, and eventually to weekly therapy with school-based support. Each setting played a important role in his recovery, but the key was ensuring smooth transitions and consistent communication between providers. Two years later, Jake serves as a peer mentor for other teenagers entering mental health treatment, helping them understand what to expect and offering hope for recovery.

His story shows how a well-coordinated system of care can provide the right services at the right time, supporting children and families through their most difficult moments while building on their strengths and resilience. When we get this coordination right, we don't just treat mental illness—we help children and families thrive.

Chapter 14: Legal, Ethical, and Regulatory Considerations

Sixteen-year-old Marcus sat across from his therapist, tears streaming down his face as he described feeling hopeless about his future. Then he said the words that made the therapist's stomach drop: "I've been thinking about killing myself. I have a plan, and I know when I want to do it."

The therapist faced a dilemma that pediatric mental health providers encounter regularly. Marcus was a minor who'd been coming to therapy with his parents' knowledge, but he'd specifically asked that this information not be shared with them. He was old enough to understand the consequences of his thoughts but still legally a child. The therapist needed to balance Marcus's right to confidentiality with the duty to protect him from harm, all while considering his parents' rights and responsibilities.

These situations highlight the complex legal and ethical terrain that pediatric mental health providers must navigate daily. Unlike adult mental health services, working with minors involves additional layers of complexity around consent, confidentiality, mandatory reporting, and decision-making authority. Understanding these legal and ethical frameworks isn't just about avoiding lawsuits—it's about providing ethical, effective care while protecting both children and families.

The Legal Foundations

The legal framework governing pediatric mental health services involves federal laws, state statutes, professional regulations, and court decisions that together create a complex web of requirements and protections.

Federal Legal Framework

Health Insurance Portability and Accountability Act (HIPAA): HIPAA protects the privacy of health information, including mental health records. However, when minors are involved, the picture becomes more complicated because parents typically have rights to access their children's health information.

Family Educational Rights and Privacy Act (FERPA): FERPA governs the privacy of educational records, which can include mental health information when services are provided in schools.

Emergency Medical Treatment and Labor Act (EMTALA): EMTALA requires hospitals to provide emergency screening and stabilization, including psychiatric emergencies, regardless of ability to pay.

Americans with Disabilities Act (ADA) and Section 504: These laws prohibit discrimination based on mental health conditions and may require accommodations in schools and other settings.

State Law Variations

Mental health laws vary significantly from state to state, creating challenges for providers who work across state lines or for families who move. Key areas of variation include:

Age of Consent for Mental Health Treatment:

- Some states allow minors as young as 12 to consent to mental health treatment
- Others require parental consent until age 18
- Many states have exceptions for specific situations like substance abuse or sexual assault

Confidentiality Protections:

- Different rules about what information can be shared with parents
- Varying requirements for obtaining minor consent before sharing information
- Different standards for when confidentiality can be breached

Mandatory Reporting Requirements:

- All states require reporting of suspected child abuse
- Different definitions of what constitutes abuse or neglect
- Varying requirements for reporting other situations like suicidal ideation

Consent and Assent in Pediatric Mental Health

Understanding consent and assent is crucial for anyone working with minors in mental health settings.

Legal Consent vs. Informed Assent

Consent: Legal authorization for treatment given by someone with legal authority to make healthcare decisions. For minors, this is typically parents or legal guardians.

Assent: Agreement to treatment given by a minor who may not have legal authority but has sufficient understanding to participate in treatment decisions.

Age-Based Considerations

Early Childhood (Ages 2-7):

- Parents provide consent for all treatment decisions
- Children may give simple assent for specific activities ("Is it okay if we play with these toys today?")
- Focus on building trust and cooperation rather than formal decision-making

School Age (Ages 8-12):

- Parents continue to provide legal consent
- Children can provide more meaningful assent and should be included in age-appropriate discussions
- Begin introducing concepts of confidentiality and privacy

Adolescence (Ages 13-18):

- Legal consent requirements vary by state
- Adolescents can provide meaningful assent and should be included in treatment planning
- Balancing adolescent autonomy with parental rights becomes more complex

Mature Minor Doctrine

Some states recognize the "mature minor" doctrine, which allows adolescents to make certain healthcare decisions if they demonstrate sufficient maturity and understanding. Factors considered include:

- Age and maturity level
- Understanding of treatment risks and benefits
- Ability to make reasoned decisions
- Complexity and risk level of proposed treatment

Emancipated Minors

Minors who are legally emancipated (through marriage, military service, court order, or financial independence) can generally consent to their own mental health treatment. However, the requirements for emancipation vary by state.

Special Consent Situations

Emergency Treatment: When immediate treatment is necessary to prevent serious harm, providers can typically provide emergency mental health services without parental consent.

Specific Conditions: Many states allow minors to consent to treatment for specific conditions like:

- Substance abuse
- Sexual assault
- Pregnancy-related services
- Sexually transmitted infections

Consider Sarah, a 15-year-old who seeks therapy after being sexually assaulted. Her state allows minors to consent to mental health treatment related to sexual abuse without parental involvement. Sarah can legally consent to therapy, but her therapist still needs to consider whether involving parents would be helpful or harmful to her recovery.

Confidentiality with Minors

Confidentiality in pediatric mental health involves balancing multiple competing interests: the child's privacy rights, parents' rights to information about their child, and the need to protect children from harm.

HIPAA and Minors

HIPAA generally allows parents to access their minor children's health information, but there are several important exceptions:

State Law Exceptions: When state laws give minors the right to consent to treatment, parents may not have automatic access to that information.

Provider Discretion: HIPAA allows (but doesn't require) providers to use professional judgment about whether sharing information with parents would be in the child's best interest.

Adolescent Request: Some providers honor adolescents' requests for confidentiality even when not legally required to do so.

Therapeutic Confidentiality

Beyond legal requirements, maintaining appropriate confidentiality is essential for building therapeutic relationships with children and adolescents.

Building Trust: Children need to know they can share sensitive information without it automatically being shared with parents.

Age-Appropriate Boundaries: Confidentiality boundaries should match children's developmental level and the nature of information shared.

Family Dynamics: Providers must consider how sharing or not sharing information might affect family relationships.

Common Confidentiality Dilemmas

Minor Reports Substance Use: A 16-year-old tells their therapist about occasional marijuana use. Should this information be shared with parents?

Adolescent Sexual Activity: A 15-year-old discusses being sexually active with their boyfriend. Are parents entitled to this information?

Family Conflict: A 14-year-old shares frustration about strict parents and expresses wishes to live with grandparents. How much should be shared with parents?

Best Practices for Managing Confidentiality

Upfront Discussions: At the beginning of treatment, discuss confidentiality policies with both parents and children in age-appropriate terms.

Written Agreements: Some providers use written agreements outlining what information will and won't be shared with parents.

Regular Check-ins: Periodically revisit confidentiality agreements as children mature and situations change.

Collaborative Approaches: When possible, help children find ways to share important information with parents themselves, with therapist support.

Documentation: Carefully document decisions about confidentiality and the reasoning behind them.

Think about Alex, a 17-year-old who reveals to their therapist that they're questioning their gender identity but aren't ready to discuss this with parents. The therapist needs to balance Alex's need for privacy and safety with the potential benefits of family support. The therapist might work with Alex over time to explore ways to share this information when Alex feels ready, while maintaining confidentiality in the meantime.

Mandatory Reporting Requirements

All mental health providers are mandated reporters, meaning they're legally required to report suspected child abuse or neglect to authorities. However, the specifics of these requirements vary by state and situation.

What Must Be Reported

Physical Abuse:

- Non-accidental injuries caused by caregivers
- Excessive or inappropriate physical discipline
- Injuries inconsistent with explanations provided

Sexual Abuse:

- Sexual contact between adults and children
- Sexual activity between children with significant age or power differences

- Exposure to inappropriate sexual material or situations

Emotional Abuse:

- Severe or persistent emotional maltreatment
- Threats, rejection, or criticism that impairs child's development
- Witnessing domestic violence (in some states)

Neglect:

- Failure to provide basic needs (food, shelter, medical care, education)
- Inadequate supervision resulting in risk of harm
- Educational neglect (chronic truancy without valid reasons)

Reporting Standards

"Reasonable Suspicion" Standard: Most states require reporting when providers have "reasonable suspicion" of abuse, not proof or certainty.

"In Good Faith" Protections: Providers who report in good faith are protected from liability, even if investigation doesn't substantiate abuse.

Failure to Report Consequences: Failing to report suspected abuse can result in criminal charges, loss of professional license, and civil liability.

Special Reporting Situations

Historical Abuse: When children report abuse that occurred in the past, reporting requirements may vary depending on:

- Whether the perpetrator still has access to children
- Whether the abuse is ongoing
- The age of the victim and perpetrator

- State-specific statutes of limitations

Peer-on-Peer Abuse: When children are abused by other minors, reporting requirements depend on:

- Age difference between children
- Nature and severity of the abuse
- Whether adequate supervision was provided

Parental Mental Illness or Substance Use: Mental health conditions or substance use alone don't constitute abuse, but may require reporting if they result in:

- Inability to provide adequate care
- Dangerous situations for children
- Neglect of basic needs

The Reporting Process

Immediate Report: Most states require immediate oral reports (within 24-48 hours) followed by written reports within a specified timeframe.

Information to Include:

- Child's name, age, and address
- Names of parents/caregivers
- Nature and extent of suspected abuse
- Evidence or observations supporting suspicion
- Reporter's name and contact information

Follow-up Responsibilities: After reporting, providers should:

- Document the report carefully
- Cooperate with investigation if requested
- Continue providing therapeutic support to the child
- Maintain appropriate boundaries with investigating agencies

Supporting Children Through Reports

Making a child abuse report can significantly impact the therapeutic relationship and the child's wellbeing.

Preparing Children: When possible, prepare children for what will happen after a report is made, including:

- Who will be contacted
- What kinds of questions they might be asked
- Their right to have support during interviews
- That the report was made to help keep them safe

Maintaining Trust:

- Explain that reporting was required by law, not a choice
- Emphasize that the child is not in trouble
- Reassure them that therapy will continue
- Address any fears or concerns they express

Ongoing Support:

- Continue providing therapeutic support throughout investigation
- Help children process their feelings about the report and investigation
- Coordinate with child protective services when appropriate
- Advocate for the child's needs within the system

Consider Maria, an 8-year-old who tells her school counselor that her stepfather has been touching her inappropriately. The counselor must immediately report this to child protective services while also providing emotional support to Maria. The counselor explains in age-appropriate terms that she needs to tell some people who can help keep Maria safe, and that Maria did the right thing by telling a trusted adult.

Additional Reporting Requirements

Beyond child abuse, mental health providers may have other reporting obligations depending on state laws and specific circumstances.

Duty to Warn/Protect

Following the landmark Tarasoff case, many states have laws requiring mental health providers to warn potential victims when clients make credible threats of violence.

Requirements Typically Include:

- Identifiable victim
- Imminent threat of serious harm
- Client has means to carry out threat
- Attempts to address threat therapeutically have been insufficient

Actions May Include:

- Warning the intended victim
- Notifying law enforcement
- Involuntary hospitalization
- Other steps to protect potential victims

Suicidal Ideation Reporting

While suicidal thoughts alone don't typically require reporting to authorities, providers must take action to ensure safety:

Assessment Requirements:

- Evaluate immediate risk level
- Assess protective factors
- Determine need for increased support or supervision

Possible Interventions:

- Safety planning with client and family
- Increased session frequency
- Involvement of family or other supports
- Voluntary or involuntary hospitalization
- Removal of means of self-harm

Elder Abuse and Vulnerable Adult Reporting

When working with adolescents who are approaching adulthood, providers should be aware of vulnerable adult reporting requirements that may apply to clients with developmental disabilities or other conditions that affect capacity.

Involuntary Treatment and Hospitalization

Sometimes children need mental health treatment against their will or the will of their parents. Understanding the legal framework for involuntary treatment is crucial for protecting both children's rights and safety.

Criteria for Involuntary Hospitalization

Most states allow involuntary psychiatric hospitalization of minors when:

- They pose immediate danger to themselves or others
- They're gravely disabled and unable to care for basic needs
- They need treatment to prevent serious deterioration

Due Process Protections

Right to Hearing: Minors (or their representatives) have the right to challenge involuntary hospitalization in court.

Legal Representation: Children have the right to legal counsel during involuntary commitment proceedings.

Independent Evaluation: Courts may order independent psychiatric evaluations to assess the need for continued involuntary treatment.

Periodic Review: Involuntary commitments must be reviewed regularly to determine if continued hospitalization is necessary.

Parental Rights vs. Child Rights

When parents and adolescents disagree about the need for mental health treatment, courts must balance:

- Parental rights to make medical decisions
- Children's rights to have their preferences considered
- State interest in protecting children's welfare
- Least restrictive treatment principles

Think about Jordan, a 16-year-old with severe anorexia whose parents want them hospitalized for medical stabilization, but Jordan refuses treatment. The treatment team must balance Jordan's autonomy and body integrity rights with the parents' authority and the medical necessity of preventing serious harm or death.

Informed Consent for Treatment

Obtaining truly informed consent for mental health treatment involves more than just getting signatures on forms. It requires ensuring that decision-makers understand the nature, risks, benefits, and alternatives to proposed treatments.

Elements of Informed Consent

Nature of Treatment:

- What specific treatments are being proposed
- How treatments work and what they involve
- Expected duration and frequency of treatment
- Goals and expected outcomes

Risks and Benefits:

- Potential positive outcomes of treatment
- Possible negative effects or side effects
- Risks of not receiving treatment
- Comparison with alternative treatments

Alternatives:

- Other treatment options available
- Consequences of choosing different treatments
- Option of no treatment and its implications

Questions and Understanding:

- Opportunity to ask questions
- Confirmation that information is understood
- Time to consider decision without pressure

Special Considerations for Minors

Developmental Understanding: Children's ability to understand treatment information varies greatly by age, maturity, and individual circumstances.

Family Dynamics: Parents and children may have different preferences or understanding of treatment needs.

Cultural Factors: Families' cultural backgrounds may influence their understanding of mental health and treatment options.

Language Barriers: When families don't speak English fluently, informed consent must be obtained in their preferred language.

Psychotropic Medications

Informed consent for psychiatric medications requires special attention to:

- FDA approval status for pediatric use (many medications are prescribed off-label)
- Black box warnings and other safety concerns
- Long-term effects that may not be fully known
- Impact on developing brains and bodies
- Need for ongoing monitoring and potential side effects

Consider the case of 12-year-old David, whose parents are considering medication for his severe ADHD. The psychiatrist must explain that while stimulant medications are well-studied in children, there are potential side effects including appetite suppression, sleep difficulties, and possible impacts on growth. The family needs to understand both the benefits of improved attention and academic performance and the risks of medication treatment.

Documentation and Record-Keeping

Proper documentation protects both providers and clients while ensuring continuity of care and legal compliance.

Legal Requirements for Records

Retention Periods: States have different requirements for how long mental health records must be maintained, typically ranging from 5-10 years after treatment ends or until the client reaches a certain age.

Content Requirements: Records must generally include:

- Assessment and diagnostic information
- Treatment plans and progress notes
- Medication records and monitoring
- Consent forms and releases of information
- Communication with other providers or agencies
- Documentation of any reporting made

Access Rights:

- Clients (or parents of minors) generally have rights to access their records
- Some states allow providers to withhold portions of records if sharing would be harmful
- Providers must respond to record requests within specified timeframes

Best Practices for Documentation

Contemporaneous Notes: Document sessions and important events as close to when they occur as possible.

Objective and Professional Language: Use factual, non-judgmental language that focuses on observations rather than interpretations.

Confidentiality Protection: Store records securely and limit access to authorized personnel only.

Error Corrections: Make corrections to records properly by drawing a single line through errors and initialing changes (never use correction fluid or delete electronic entries).

Thoroughness vs. Brevity: Include enough detail to support treatment decisions and legal protections without unnecessary information.

Electronic Health Records (EHR) Considerations

Security Requirements: Electronic records must meet HIPAA security standards including encryption, access controls, and audit trails.

Backup and Recovery: Systems must have appropriate backup and disaster recovery procedures.

User Training: Staff must be trained on proper use of EHR systems and security protocols.

Integration Challenges: When multiple providers use different systems, ensuring information sharing while maintaining security can be challenging.

Ethical Decision-Making Frameworks

When legal requirements don't provide clear guidance, ethical principles can help guide decision-making in complex situations.

Core Ethical Principles

Beneficence: Acting in the client's best interest and promoting their wellbeing.

Non-maleficence: "Do no harm" - avoiding actions that could cause damage to clients.

Autonomy: Respecting clients' rights to make decisions about their own treatment (modified for minors based on developmental capacity).

Justice: Fair and equitable treatment regardless of background, culture, or socioeconomic status.

Fidelity: Being trustworthy and honoring commitments made to clients.

Ethical Decision-Making Process

When facing ethical dilemmas:

1. **Identify the Problem:** What ethical issues are involved? Who are the stakeholders?
2. **Gather Information:** What are the relevant facts? What do professional codes of ethics say? What are the legal requirements?
3. **Consider Options:** What different courses of action are possible? What are the likely consequences of each?

4. **Apply Ethical Principles:** How do core ethical principles apply to this situation? Which principles conflict with each other?
5. **Consult Others:** Seek guidance from supervisors, colleagues, ethics committees, or professional organizations.
6. **Make and Document Decision:** Choose the course of action that best balances ethical principles and document the reasoning.
7. **Evaluate Outcomes:** After taking action, evaluate the results and learn from the experience.

Common Ethical Dilemmas

Confidentiality vs. Safety: When a teenager shares information that suggests risk but asks that it not be shared with parents.

Family vs. Individual Treatment Goals: When parents and children have different ideas about treatment goals or success.

Cultural Values vs. Professional Standards: When families' cultural or religious beliefs conflict with recommended treatments.

Resource Limitations: When ideal treatments aren't available due to insurance limitations or lack of services.

Think about the case of 15-year-old Ahmed, whose parents want him in therapy to "fix" his sexual orientation after he came out as gay. The therapist must balance respect for family values with professional ethics that prohibit conversion therapy and require affirming care for LGBTQ+ youth.

Professional Liability and Risk Management

Understanding liability risks and implementing appropriate risk management strategies protects both providers and the clients they serve.

Common Liability Risks

Failure to Assess Suicide Risk: Inadequate assessment or response to suicidal ideation is one of the most common sources of malpractice claims.

Breach of Confidentiality: Inappropriate sharing of client information, whether intentional or accidental, can result in legal action.

Failure to Report Abuse: Not reporting suspected child abuse when required by law can result in both criminal charges and civil liability.

Practicing Outside Competence: Providing services without adequate training or experience can result in harm to clients and professional liability.

Boundary Violations: Inappropriate relationships or interactions with clients can lead to professional discipline and legal action.

Risk Management Strategies

Professional Liability Insurance: Carry adequate malpractice insurance that covers both claims and regulatory investigations.

Continuing Education: Stay current on legal requirements, ethical guidelines, and best practices through ongoing training.

Consultation and Supervision: Regularly consult with colleagues and supervisors about challenging cases and ethical dilemmas.

Documentation: Maintain thorough, accurate records that support treatment decisions and demonstrate adherence to standards of care.

Informed Consent: Ensure clients understand treatments, risks, and alternatives before beginning services.

Scope of Practice: Stay within areas of competence and refer clients to other providers when appropriate.

Working with Special Populations

Certain populations of children present unique legal and ethical considerations that require specialized knowledge and approaches.

Children in Foster Care

Consent Issues: Determine who has legal authority to consent to mental health treatment (biological parents, foster parents, caseworkers, or courts).

Information Sharing: Understand requirements for sharing information with caseworkers, attorneys, and courts while protecting appropriate confidentiality.

Placement Stability: Consider how treatment recommendations might affect placement decisions and child's overall wellbeing.

Justice-Involved Youth

Confidentiality Limitations: Understand how involvement with probation or courts affects confidentiality protections.

Competency Evaluations: Be aware of requirements for assessing youth competency to stand trial or waive rights.

Treatment vs. Punishment: Navigate tensions between therapeutic goals and legal system requirements.

Children with Developmental Disabilities

Capacity Assessment: Evaluate children's capacity to participate in treatment decisions based on their individual abilities rather than chronological age.

Guardianship Issues: Understand when parents retain decision-making authority versus when guardians are appointed.

Advocacy Needs: Consider additional advocacy that may be needed to ensure appropriate services and protections.

Quality Assurance and Regulatory Compliance

Mental health organizations must implement systems to ensure ongoing compliance with legal requirements and quality standards.

Regulatory Bodies

State Licensing Boards: Regulate individual professional licenses and investigate complaints about professional conduct.

State Health Departments: May regulate mental health facilities and programs through licensing and certification requirements.

Accreditation Organizations: Organizations like The Joint Commission or CARF provide voluntary accreditation that demonstrates quality standards.

Insurance Companies: May have their own requirements for providers and facilities serving their members.

Compliance Programs

Policy Development: Organizations need comprehensive policies addressing legal requirements, ethical standards, and quality care.

Staff Training: Regular training on legal requirements, ethical guidelines, and organizational policies.

Quality Monitoring: Systems for monitoring compliance with standards and identifying areas for improvement.

Incident Reporting: Procedures for reporting and investigating adverse events or potential violations.

Corrective Action: Processes for addressing identified problems and preventing future occurrences.

Technology and Legal Considerations

The increasing use of technology in mental health services creates new legal and ethical challenges that providers must understand.

Telehealth Legal Requirements

Licensing: Providers must be licensed in the state where the client is located during telehealth sessions.

Informed Consent: Special consent requirements for telehealth services, including discussion of technology risks and limitations.

Privacy and Security: Technology platforms must meet HIPAA requirements for protecting health information.

Emergency Procedures: Clear protocols for handling mental health emergencies during telehealth sessions.

Digital Records and Communications

Secure Communication: Email, text messages, and other electronic communications with clients must be secure and HIPAA-compliant.

Social Media: Clear policies about professional use of social media and contact with clients through social platforms.

Mobile Apps: Understanding privacy policies and data security for mental health apps recommended to clients.

Building Ethical Practice

Creating and maintaining ethical practice requires ongoing attention and commitment from individuals and organizations.

Personal Ethical Development

Self-Awareness: Regular self-examination of values, biases, and potential conflicts of interest.

Professional Development: Ongoing education about legal requirements, ethical standards, and best practices.

Peer Consultation: Regular consultation with colleagues about challenging ethical issues.

Personal Therapy: Many providers find their own therapy helpful for maintaining perspective and addressing personal issues that might affect professional practice.

Organizational Ethics

Ethical Climate: Organizations should foster environments where ethical concerns can be raised and addressed openly.

Ethics Committees: Formal structures for discussing ethical dilemmas and developing organizational policies.

Leadership Modeling: Leaders should demonstrate ethical behavior and support staff in making ethical decisions.

System Supports: Providing resources, training, and support needed for staff to practice ethically.

Putting It All Together

The legal and ethical aspects of pediatric mental health practice can seem overwhelming, but they all serve the same fundamental purpose: protecting children while providing effective, ethical care.

Marcus, the suicidal teenager from our opening example, represents the complexity these issues create in real practice. His therapist had to quickly consider multiple factors: Marcus's safety, his right to confidentiality, his parents' rights and concerns, legal reporting requirements, and ethical obligations.

The therapist decided to work with Marcus to develop a safety plan and helped him find ways to communicate his struggles to his parents with therapeutic support. This approach honored Marcus's developmental autonomy while ensuring his safety and maintaining the therapeutic relationship. The therapist documented the decision-making process carefully and consulted with a supervisor to ensure all legal and ethical obligations were met.

This case shows how legal and ethical requirements aren't barriers to good care—they're frameworks that help us provide better, safer services. When we understand these requirements and integrate them thoughtfully into our practice, we can focus on what matters most: helping children and families heal and thrive.

The legal and ethical landscape will continue to evolve as technology advances, social attitudes change, and new research emerges. Staying current with these changes isn't just a professional obligation—it's an opportunity to continuously improve the quality and effectiveness of the care we provide.

Chapter 15: Technology and Innovation in Pediatric Mental Health

Thirteen-year-old Zoe stared at her smartphone screen at 11:30 PM, tears streaming down her face. She'd been having panic attacks for weeks but felt too embarrassed to tell her parents. A quick Google search led her to a mental health app that promised to help with anxiety. Within minutes, she was practicing breathing exercises and learning about what panic attacks actually were. For the first time in weeks, she didn't feel completely alone.

Meanwhile, across the country, 16-year-old Carlos was in his weekly therapy session—but instead of sitting in an office, he was at home talking to his therapist through a secure video platform. Living in a rural area with no mental health professionals nearby, telehealth had become his lifeline to getting the support he needed.

These stories reflect a rapidly changing reality in pediatric mental health. Technology is transforming how we identify, assess, and treat mental health challenges in children and adolescents. Digital tools are making services more accessible, engaging, and personalized than ever before. But with these opportunities come new challenges around safety, privacy, effectiveness, and the digital divide.

The Digital Generation and Mental Health

Today's children and adolescents are true digital natives. They've grown up with smartphones, social media, and instant connectivity. This reality creates both opportunities and challenges for mental health care.

Digital Native Characteristics

Always Connected: Most teenagers are online almost constantly, with 95% having access to a smartphone and 45% reporting they're online "almost constantly."

Comfort with Technology: Young people often prefer digital communication and may feel more comfortable expressing difficult emotions through technology than face-to-face.

Information Seeking: When facing challenges, many youth turn to the internet first for information and support.

Peer Networks: Social connections often happen online, making digital platforms important spaces for both support and potential harm.

Mental Health Implications

Increased Help-Seeking: Technology can lower barriers to seeking information and support about mental health challenges.

Reduced Stigma: Anonymous or private digital tools may feel less stigmatizing than traditional mental health services.

24/7 Access: Digital tools can provide support and resources when traditional services aren't available.

Personalization: Technology allows for customized interventions that adapt to individual needs and preferences.

But technology also creates new mental health risks:

Social Media Pressure: Constant comparison with others and pressure to present a perfect online image can contribute to anxiety and depression.

Cyberbullying: Online harassment can be particularly devastating because it follows children home and can happen 24/7.

Sleep Disruption: Screen time, especially before bed, can interfere with sleep patterns that are crucial for mental health.

Reduced Face-to-Face Interaction: Over-reliance on digital communication may impact social skill development and emotional intelligence.

Telehealth in Pediatric Mental Health

The COVID-19 pandemic accelerated the adoption of telehealth services, demonstrating both their potential and their limitations.

Types of Telehealth Services

Synchronous Video Sessions: Real-time video conversations between providers and clients, most similar to traditional in-person therapy.

Asynchronous Communication: Secure messaging, email exchanges, or recorded video messages that don't require both parties to be online simultaneously.

Hybrid Models: Combinations of in-person and virtual sessions that maximize the benefits of both approaches.

Group Telehealth: Virtual group therapy sessions that can connect youth with similar challenges regardless of geographic location.

Effectiveness of Telehealth

Research has consistently shown that telehealth can be as effective as in-person treatment for many mental health conditions:

Depression and Anxiety: Multiple studies have found equivalent outcomes for depression and anxiety treatment delivered via telehealth versus in-person.

ADHD Management: Telehealth has proven effective for ADHD assessment, medication management, and parent training.

Autism Services: Parent training and behavioral interventions for children with autism can be effectively delivered through telehealth.

Crisis Services: Text and video crisis counseling services have shown effectiveness in reducing immediate distress and connecting youth to ongoing services.

Benefits of Telehealth for Young People

Accessibility: Eliminates transportation barriers and makes services available in underserved areas.

Flexibility: Sessions can be scheduled more easily around school and family obligations.

Comfort: Some youth feel more comfortable in their own environment and may be more open in virtual sessions.

Continuity: Treatment can continue despite illness, weather, family crises, or other disruptions.

Family Involvement: Easier to include family members in sessions when everyone is already at home.

Challenges and Limitations

Technology Barriers: Not all families have reliable internet access or appropriate devices for video sessions.

Privacy Concerns: Ensuring privacy during home-based sessions can be challenging in crowded living situations.

Therapeutic Relationship: Building rapport and connection may be more difficult through a screen, especially with younger children.

Crisis Management: Handling mental health emergencies is more complex when the therapist and client are in different locations.

Nonverbal Communication: Limited ability to observe body language and nonverbal cues that are important in therapy.

Best Practices for Telehealth with Youth

Environmental Setup:

- Encourage private, quiet spaces for sessions
- Ensure good lighting and camera positioning
- Have backup communication plans if technology fails

Engagement Strategies:

- Use interactive features like screen sharing and virtual whiteboards
- Incorporate movement and activities appropriate for virtual format
- Keep sessions slightly shorter than in-person meetings, especially for younger children

Family Involvement:

- Be intentional about when family members should and shouldn't be present
- Use separate devices or rooms when individual privacy is needed
- Include family members in ways that support rather than interfere with treatment

Safety Planning:

- Know local emergency resources near client's location

- Have clear protocols for handling crises during virtual sessions
- Maintain updated emergency contact information

Consider Emma, a 14-year-old with social anxiety who initially refused to attend in-person therapy because she was terrified of meeting new people. Through telehealth, she was able to begin treatment in the comfort of her own room. After building a strong therapeutic relationship virtually, she eventually felt confident enough to transition to in-person sessions.

Digital Mental Health Tools and Applications

The digital health market includes thousands of apps and online programs claiming to support mental health. While many show promise, the quality and effectiveness vary dramatically.

Categories of Digital Mental Health Tools

Mood Tracking Apps: Help users monitor their emotional states, identify patterns, and track progress over time.

Meditation and Mindfulness Apps: Provide guided meditations, breathing exercises, and mindfulness practices.

Cognitive Behavioral Therapy (CBT) Apps: Interactive programs that teach CBT skills and techniques for managing anxiety, depression, and other conditions.

Crisis Support Apps: Provide immediate access to crisis resources, safety planning tools, and emergency contacts.

Educational Apps: Offer information about mental health conditions, coping strategies, and recovery resources.

Peer Support Platforms: Connect users with others facing similar challenges for mutual support and encouragement.

Evidence-Based Digital Interventions

While most mental health apps lack rigorous research support, several have demonstrated effectiveness in clinical trials:

SPARX: A gaming-based CBT intervention for adolescents with depression that has shown effectiveness in multiple studies.

MindShift: An anxiety management app based on CBT principles that has research support for reducing anxiety symptoms.

Sanvello: Combines mood tracking, CBT techniques, and peer support with evidence showing reductions in anxiety and depression.

Crisis Text Line: Text-based crisis counseling service with research demonstrating effectiveness in de-escalating crises.

Benefits of Digital Mental Health Tools

24/7 Availability: Support and resources are available whenever youth need them, including nights and weekends.

Privacy and Anonymity: Many tools can be used privately without others knowing, reducing stigma barriers.

Engagement: Interactive features, games, and personalized content can be more engaging than traditional educational materials.

Cost-Effectiveness: Many apps are free or low-cost, making them accessible to families with limited resources.

Skill Building: Apps can provide structured skill-building exercises and practice opportunities between therapy sessions.

Risks and Limitations

Limited Evidence: Most mental health apps haven't been rigorously tested for safety or effectiveness.

Privacy Concerns: Many apps collect personal data that may not be adequately protected or may be shared with third parties.

Inappropriate Content: Some apps may provide inaccurate information or recommend strategies that could be harmful.

Over-reliance: Apps shouldn't replace professional treatment for serious mental health conditions.

Digital Divide: Not all youth have access to smartphones or internet connectivity needed to use digital tools.

Evaluating Digital Mental Health Tools

When considering apps or digital tools, important factors to evaluate include:

Evidence Base: Is there research supporting the app's effectiveness? Has it been tested with the target population?

Clinical Oversight: Are mental health professionals involved in developing and monitoring the app?

Privacy Policy: How is user data collected, stored, and shared? Are there adequate privacy protections?

Safety Features: Does the app have appropriate safety measures for users in crisis? Are there clear limitations and when to seek professional help?

User Experience: Is the app easy to use and engaging? Does it provide helpful features without being overwhelming?

Cost and Sustainability: What are the costs, both upfront and ongoing? Will the app continue to be supported and updated?

Integration: Can the app work alongside professional treatment? Does it allow for sharing data with healthcare providers when appropriate?

Think about Tyler, a 15-year-old who downloaded a popular mood tracking app after feeling depressed. The app helped him notice that his mood dipped significantly on Sundays (when he worried about the upcoming school week) and improved after exercise. This self-awareness helped him develop coping strategies and gave him concrete information to share with his therapist.

Social Media Impact on Youth Mental Health

Social media platforms have become central to how young people communicate, form identity, and understand the world around them. Understanding these impacts is crucial for mental health providers.

The Scope of Social Media Use

Nearly Universal Adoption: 95% of teens have access to a smartphone, and 72% check for social media messages or notifications as soon as they wake up.

Platform Diversity: Different platforms serve different purposes - Instagram for visual content, Snapchat for ephemeral messaging, TikTok for short videos, Discord for gaming communities.

Time Investment: Teens spend an average of 7-9 hours daily on various media, with a significant portion on social platforms.

Positive Impacts on Mental Health

Social Connection: Social media helps youth maintain friendships and connect with others who share similar interests or challenges.

Identity Exploration: Platforms provide spaces for youth to explore different aspects of their identity and connect with communities that affirm their experiences.

Mental Health Resources: Many young people discover mental health information, resources, and support through social media platforms.

Creative Expression: Platforms provide outlets for artistic expression, storytelling, and sharing creative work.

Crisis Support: Youth may reach out for help through social media when they wouldn't access traditional services.

Negative Impacts on Mental Health

Social Comparison: Constant exposure to others' highlight reels can increase feelings of inadequacy and lower self-esteem.

Cyberbullying: Online harassment can be particularly damaging because it follows youth home and can involve public humiliation.

Sleep Disruption: Late-night social media use interferes with sleep patterns that are crucial for mental health.

Fear of Missing Out (FOMO): Seeing others' activities can increase anxiety and feelings of social exclusion.

Echo Chambers: Algorithms may reinforce negative thinking patterns or expose youth to harmful content.

Platform-Specific Considerations

Instagram: Visual focus can increase body image concerns and social comparison, but also provides platforms for mental health advocacy and education.

TikTok: Short-form videos can spread mental health awareness quickly but may also normalize or romanticize mental illness.

Snapchat: Disappearing messages can facilitate risky behavior, but streaks and scores can create pressure to maintain constant contact.

Discord: Gaming-focused communities can provide strong social support but may also expose youth to inappropriate content or predatory behavior.

Helping Youth Navigate Social Media Safely

Digital Literacy: Teaching critical thinking about online content, including recognizing manipulation and misinformation.

Privacy Settings: Understanding how to control who can see posts and personal information.

Time Management: Developing healthy boundaries around social media use, including breaks and offline time.

Curating Feeds: Actively choosing to follow accounts that are positive and supportive rather than those that trigger negative feelings.

Reporting and Blocking: Knowing how to respond to cyberbullying, inappropriate contact, or harmful content.

Consider Jasmine, a 16-year-old who developed an eating disorder partly influenced by "thinspiration" content she encountered on Instagram. Her therapist helped her understand how algorithms had created a harmful echo chamber and worked with her to curate a feed filled with body-positive content and recovery resources. This shift in her social media environment became an important part of her healing process.

Artificial Intelligence and Machine Learning

AI and machine learning technologies are beginning to transform how mental health services are delivered, from screening and assessment to treatment and monitoring.

AI in Mental Health Screening

Natural Language Processing: AI can analyze text from social media posts, online surveys, or therapy notes to identify language patterns associated with depression, anxiety, or suicidal ideation.

Voice Analysis: Changes in speech patterns, tone, and vocal characteristics may indicate mood changes or mental health concerns.

Behavioral Analysis: Smartphone sensors can track patterns in movement, sleep, social interaction, and app usage that may correlate with mental health symptoms.

Image Analysis: AI can analyze facial expressions in photos or videos to assess emotional states over time.

AI-Powered Interventions

Chatbots and Virtual Therapists: AI-powered chatbots can provide 24/7 support, basic counseling techniques, and crisis intervention.

Personalized Treatment: Machine learning can analyze large datasets to predict which treatments are most likely to be effective for individual patients.

Real-Time Monitoring: AI can continuously monitor symptoms and alert providers when intervention may be needed.

Automated Check-ins: AI systems can conduct regular assessments and follow-ups, freeing human providers to focus on complex cases.

Benefits of AI in Mental Health

Accessibility: AI tools can provide basic mental health support in areas with provider shortages.

Early Detection: Continuous monitoring may identify mental health concerns before they become severe.

Personalization: AI can tailor interventions to individual needs and preferences in ways that wouldn't be feasible manually.

Cost-Effectiveness: AI tools may reduce costs while maintaining quality of care for certain types of interventions.

Objectivity: AI assessments may be less subject to human bias in diagnosis and treatment recommendations.

Limitations and Concerns

Limited Understanding: AI lacks the nuanced understanding of human experience that's crucial for mental health care.

Data Privacy: AI systems often require large amounts of personal data, raising significant privacy concerns.

Bias and Fairness: AI systems can perpetuate or amplify existing biases in healthcare, particularly affecting marginalized communities.

Regulation and Oversight: Limited regulatory frameworks for AI mental health tools raise safety and quality concerns.

Human Connection: AI cannot replace the therapeutic relationship and human connection that are central to mental health healing.

Current Examples of AI in Practice

Woebot: An AI-powered chatbot that provides CBT-based interventions and has shown effectiveness in reducing symptoms of depression and anxiety.

Wysa: An AI companion that provides emotional support and teaches coping skills, particularly popular among teenagers.

X2AI: Platform that uses AI to match clients with appropriate human therapists and provides AI-assisted therapy sessions.

Ellipsis Health: Uses voice analysis to screen for depression and anxiety, with potential applications in healthcare settings.

Virtual and Augmented Reality in Mental Health

Immersive technologies are opening new possibilities for mental health treatment, particularly for anxiety disorders, PTSD, and social skills training.

Virtual Reality Applications

Exposure Therapy: VR can create controlled environments for gradual exposure to feared situations, such as heights, social situations, or trauma-related triggers.

Relaxation and Mindfulness: Immersive environments can enhance meditation and relaxation exercises by providing calming, distraction-free spaces.

Social Skills Training: VR can provide safe environments for practicing social interactions, particularly beneficial for youth with autism or social anxiety.

Pain Management: VR distraction techniques can help manage pain during medical procedures or chronic pain conditions.

Augmented Reality Applications

Real-Time Support: AR can overlay coping strategies or calming techniques onto real-world environments during stressful situations.

Educational Tools: AR can make mental health education more engaging and interactive.

Biofeedback: AR can provide real-time feedback about physiological states like heart rate or breathing patterns.

Benefits for Youth

Engagement: Immersive technologies may be more engaging than traditional therapeutic activities, particularly for digital natives.

Safety: VR provides controlled environments where youth can practice skills or face fears without real-world consequences.

Accessibility: Once developed, VR interventions can be delivered in various settings without requiring specialized therapist training.

Consistency: VR environments provide standardized experiences that can be replicated exactly across different sessions or users.

Challenges and Limitations

Cost: VR equipment and software development require significant initial investments.

Technical Issues: Equipment malfunctions or technical difficulties can disrupt therapeutic sessions.

Motion Sickness: Some users experience nausea or discomfort when using VR, particularly during longer sessions.

Limited Applications: VR is most effective for specific types of interventions and may not be suitable for all mental health conditions.

Therapist Training: Providers need training to effectively incorporate VR into therapeutic practice.

Think about Marcus, a 17-year-old with severe social anxiety who avoided group situations and had difficulty making friends. His therapist used VR to help him practice conversations in various social settings - cafeterias, parties, job interviews. The safe, controlled environment allowed Marcus to build confidence and skills before applying them in real-world situations.

Gaming and Gamification in Mental Health

The popularity of gaming among youth has led to increased interest in using game-based approaches for mental health education and intervention.

Types of Mental Health Games

Serious Games: Games specifically designed for mental health education or intervention, such as SPARX for depression or MindLight for anxiety.

Gamified Apps: Traditional mental health tools that incorporate game elements like points, levels, and rewards.

Commercial Games: Existing commercial games that may have therapeutic benefits, such as puzzle games for cognitive training or social games for connection.

Virtual Worlds: Immersive online environments where youth can interact with others and practice social skills.

Benefits of Gaming Approaches

Engagement: Games can make mental health interventions more engaging and enjoyable, increasing participation and completion rates.

Skill Practice: Games provide opportunities to practice coping skills and strategies in low-stakes environments.

Immediate Feedback: Games can provide instant feedback on performance and progress.

Motivation: Game mechanics like achievements and progress tracking can increase motivation to continue with interventions.

Peer Connection: Multiplayer games can facilitate social connections and peer support.

Considerations and Limitations

Quality Variation: The quality and evidence base for mental health games varies significantly.

Screen Time Concerns: Adding games to mental health treatment may increase overall screen time exposure.

Gaming Addiction: Some youth may be vulnerable to problematic gaming behaviors.

Superficial Engagement: Game elements alone don't guarantee meaningful therapeutic engagement.

Cost and Access: High-quality therapeutic games may be expensive and not accessible to all families.

Digital Divide and Equity Considerations

While technology offers tremendous opportunities for expanding mental health services, it also risks creating new forms of inequality if not implemented thoughtfully.

Dimensions of the Digital Divide

Access to Devices: Not all families can afford smartphones, tablets, or computers needed for digital mental health services.

Internet Connectivity: Reliable high-speed internet isn't available in all communities, particularly rural and low-income areas.

Digital Literacy: Comfort and skill with technology varies significantly among different populations.

Language Barriers: Most digital mental health tools are available only in English, limiting access for non-English speaking families.

Privacy and Safety: Families may lack safe, private spaces needed for telehealth sessions or may have concerns about data privacy.

Impact on Mental Health Services

Increased Disparities: If digital tools primarily benefit families with resources and access, existing mental health disparities may widen.

Rural Communities: Areas with limited internet infrastructure may be unable to benefit from telehealth and digital interventions.

Economic Barriers: Costs of devices, internet service, and premium app features may exclude low-income families.

Cultural Relevance: Many digital tools are developed for majority populations and may not be culturally relevant for diverse communities.

Strategies for Promoting Equity

Device Lending Programs: Mental health organizations can lend tablets or smartphones to families who need them for telehealth services.

Public-Private Partnerships: Collaborations with internet service providers to expand access in underserved areas.

Multilingual Resources: Developing and translating digital mental health tools into multiple languages.

Community-Based Access: Providing telehealth services through schools, libraries, and community centers with reliable internet.

Sliding Scale Fees: Offering reduced-cost or free access to premium digital mental health tools based on family income.

Cultural Adaptation: Modifying existing tools or developing new ones that reflect diverse cultural values and experiences.

Privacy and Safety in Digital Mental Health

The digital nature of many new mental health tools creates unique privacy and safety considerations that providers and families must understand.

Data Privacy Concerns

Information Collection: Many apps collect extensive personal information, including location data, contacts, and detailed mental health information.

Data Sharing: User data may be shared with third parties for marketing, research, or other purposes without clear user understanding.

Security Breaches: Mental health data is particularly sensitive, and security breaches can have serious consequences for individuals.

Government Surveillance: Concerns about government access to mental health data, particularly for undocumented immigrants or other vulnerable populations.

Safety Considerations

Crisis Situations: Digital tools may not have adequate safety measures for users in mental health crises.

Inappropriate Content: Some platforms may expose youth to harmful content related to self-harm, suicide, or eating disorders.

Predatory Behavior: Online platforms can provide opportunities for adults to exploit or harm vulnerable youth.

Misinformation: Inaccurate mental health information can be harmful, particularly if it discourages appropriate treatment.

Best Practices for Digital Safety

Privacy Policy Review: Read and understand privacy policies before using mental health apps or platforms.

Secure Platforms: Use only HIPAA-compliant platforms for telehealth sessions.

Strong Passwords: Create strong, unique passwords for mental health-related accounts.

Regular Updates: Keep apps and devices updated with the latest security patches.

Parental Monitoring: Age-appropriate monitoring of children's digital mental health tool usage.

Professional Oversight: Involve mental health professionals in selecting and monitoring digital tools.

Emerging Technologies and Future Directions

The field of digital mental health continues to evolve rapidly, with new technologies and approaches emerging regularly.

Wearable Technology

Physiological Monitoring: Devices that track heart rate, sleep patterns, activity levels, and other indicators that may correlate with mental health.

Stress Detection: Wearables that can detect stress responses and prompt coping strategies or professional intervention.

Medication Adherence: Smart pill bottles and other devices that can track medication compliance.

Internet of Things (IoT)

Environmental Monitoring: Smart home devices that can monitor environmental factors affecting mental health, such as light exposure and air quality.

Behavioral Tracking: Connected devices that can track patterns of daily living that may indicate mental health changes.

Blockchain Technology

Data Security: Blockchain may provide more secure methods for storing and sharing mental health data.

Interoperability: Potential for creating secure, portable mental health records that patients control.

Brain-Computer Interfaces

Neurofeedback: Direct monitoring of brain activity to provide feedback for meditation, attention training, or mood regulation.

Brain Stimulation: Non-invasive brain stimulation techniques that may be controlled by computer interfaces.

Practical Implementation Guidelines

For mental health providers and organizations considering digital health tools, several practical considerations can guide implementation.

Assessment and Selection

Evidence Review: Prioritize tools with research support and avoid those with no scientific backing.

User Experience Testing: Test tools with representative users before recommending them broadly.

Integration Planning: Consider how digital tools will fit into existing treatment workflows.

Cost-Benefit Analysis: Evaluate costs against potential benefits and consider sustainability.

Training and Support

Staff Training: Ensure all staff understand how to use and troubleshoot digital tools.

Client Education: Provide comprehensive education about digital tool usage, benefits, and limitations.

Ongoing Support: Establish systems for ongoing technical support and troubleshooting.

Quality Assurance

Regular Review: Continuously evaluate the effectiveness and safety of digital tools in use.

Client Feedback: Regularly collect and act on user feedback about digital tool experiences.

Outcome Monitoring: Track clinical outcomes to ensure digital tools are supporting treatment goals.

Balancing Innovation with Human Connection

While technology offers exciting possibilities for expanding and improving mental health services, it's important to remember that healing ultimately happens in relationship.

The Irreplaceable Human Element

Empathy and Understanding: Human providers offer emotional understanding and empathy that technology cannot replicate.

Complex Problem-Solving: Mental health challenges often require nuanced understanding and creative solutions that AI cannot provide.

Ethical Decision-Making: Human judgment is essential for navigating complex ethical situations in mental health care.

Cultural Sensitivity: Human providers can understand and respond to cultural nuances that may be missed by technology.

Technology as Enhancement, Not Replacement

The most effective approach may be using technology to enhance rather than replace human connection:

Augmented Therapy: Using technology to support and extend traditional therapy rather than replacing it.

Blended Care Models: Combining in-person and digital services to maximize benefits of both approaches.

Provider Tools: Using technology to help human providers deliver more effective and efficient care.

Accessibility Bridge: Using technology to reach people who cannot access traditional services while working toward increasing human provider availability.

Technology will continue transforming pediatric mental health services, but implementation must be thoughtful and evidence-based.

Zoe and Carlos from our opening examples represent both the promise and the complexity of digital mental health. Zoe found immediate support through a mental health app when she needed it most, but she also needed guidance to ensure she was using reliable, safe resources. Carlos accessed high-quality therapy through telehealth that wouldn't have been possible otherwise, but his treatment was most effective when it included family involvement and coordination with his school.

These stories show that technology isn't magic—it's a tool that can be incredibly powerful when used appropriately. The key is ensuring that digital mental health innovations truly serve the needs of children and families rather than simply capitalizing on the latest technological trends.

As we continue developing and implementing new technologies, we must keep several principles in mind: evidence should guide adoption, equity must be prioritized, privacy and safety are non-negotiable, and human connection remains at the heart of healing.

The future of pediatric mental health will likely involve seamless integration of technology with traditional services, creating more accessible, engaging, and effective care than either approach could provide alone. But achieving this future requires careful attention to implementation, ongoing evaluation, and never losing sight of what matters most—helping children and families thrive.

Chapter 16: Professional Development and Leadership

At 27, Dr. Sarah Chen thought she had her career path figured out. Fresh from completing her psychiatric nurse practitioner program, she'd landed her dream job at a prestigious children's hospital. She was finally doing what she'd always wanted—helping kids with mental health challenges. But six months into the job, she found herself lying awake at night, replaying difficult cases and wondering if she was making any real difference.

The breaking point came on a Tuesday afternoon. After back-to-back crisis evaluations, Sarah sat in her car in the hospital parking garage and cried. She loved her patients, but the constant exposure to trauma, the overwhelming caseload, and the feeling of swimming against a system that seemed designed to fail children had left her depleted and questioning everything.

Sarah's story isn't unique. The pediatric mental health field is facing a workforce crisis, with high burnout rates, frequent turnover, and difficulty attracting new professionals. Yet it's also a field filled with opportunities for growth, leadership, and meaningful impact. The key lies in approaching this work with intentionality, building the skills and support systems needed not just to survive but to thrive while making a lasting difference in children's lives.

The Current State of the Pediatric Mental Health Workforce

Understanding the challenges facing the field helps contextualize both the difficulties and opportunities that lie ahead.

Workforce Shortage Statistics

The numbers paint a stark picture of need:

- 96% of U.S. counties lack adequate mental health prescribers for children
- Only 8% of nurse practitioner students specialize in psychiatric mental health
- 25% of current psychiatric mental health advanced practice registered nurses plan to retire within 6 years
- The average age of PMH-APRNs is 54, indicating urgent succession planning needs

Contributing Factors to Workforce Challenges

Educational Barriers:

- Limited pediatric psychiatric content in most nursing programs
- Few clinical rotation opportunities in pediatric mental health settings
- Lack of specialized textbooks and educational resources
- Faculty shortages in psychiatric nursing education

Financial Considerations:

- Student loan debt that may exceed $100,000 for advanced practice programs
- Lower reimbursement rates for mental health services compared to other medical specialties
- Limited scholarship and loan forgiveness programs specific to pediatric mental health

Work Environment Stressors:

- High acuity and complex cases
- Large caseloads with limited time per patient
- Frequent exposure to trauma and crisis situations
- Administrative burdens and insurance limitations
- Limited resources and support services

Professional Isolation:

- Few colleagues with similar training and interests
- Limited mentorship opportunities
- Geographic isolation in rural or underserved areas
- Stigma associated with mental health work

The Impact of Workforce Shortages

These shortages have real consequences for children and families:

- Longer wait times for services, sometimes months for initial appointments
- Emergency departments overwhelmed with mental health crises
- Children receiving inadequate or inappropriate care from providers without specialized training
- Families traveling long distances for services
- Higher costs due to lack of competition and limited options

Career Pathways in Pediatric Mental Health

Despite the challenges, pediatric mental health offers diverse and rewarding career opportunities across multiple settings and roles.

Direct Care Roles

Registered Nurses in Mental Health Settings:

- Inpatient psychiatric units
- Emergency department psychiatric nurses
- Community mental health centers
- School-based health centers
- Residential treatment facilities

Advanced Practice Registered Nurses:

- Psychiatric Mental Health Nurse Practitioners (PMHNP)

- Clinical Nurse Specialists in psychiatric nursing
- Family or pediatric nurse practitioners with mental health focus
- Nurse practitioners in integrated care settings

Specialized Nursing Roles:

- Forensic psychiatric nursing with justice-involved youth
- Consultation-liaison nursing in medical settings
- Addictions nursing focusing on adolescent populations
- Trauma-informed care specialists

Leadership and Administrative Roles

Clinical Leadership:

- Charge nurses and shift supervisors
- Clinical coordinators and program managers
- Quality improvement specialists
- Risk management professionals

Executive Leadership:

- Nursing directors and chief nursing officers
- Program directors for mental health services
- Chief executive officers of mental health organizations
- Chief clinical officers overseeing multiple programs

Education and Research Careers

Academic Positions:

- Faculty in nursing schools teaching psychiatric nursing
- Clinical instructors and preceptors
- Simulation lab specialists
- Curriculum developers and education consultants

Research Roles:

- Clinical researchers studying interventions and outcomes
- Health services researchers examining system improvements
- Policy researchers analyzing mental health legislation and regulations
- Nurse scientists leading interdisciplinary research teams

Entrepreneurship and Innovation

Private Practice:

- Solo or group practices providing therapy or medication management
- Consultation services to schools, organizations, or other providers
- Specialized services for specific populations or conditions

Business and Technology:

- Developing digital mental health tools and applications
- Creating educational programs and resources
- Consulting on mental health program development
- Healthcare technology companies focusing on mental health solutions

Consider Maria Rodriguez, who started as a staff nurse on a pediatric psychiatric unit. Through continuing education and leadership development, she became a clinical nurse specialist, then program director, and eventually chief nursing officer for a large mental health system. Each role built on her clinical experience while allowing her to impact more children and families through system-level improvements.

Professional Certification and Credentialing

Professional certifications demonstrate expertise and commitment while often providing career advancement opportunities and higher salaries.

Nursing Certifications

Psychiatric-Mental Health Nursing Certification:

- Basic certification for registered nurses (RN-BC)
- Advanced practice certification for nurse practitioners (PMHNP-BC)
- Offered through the American Nurses Credentialing Center (ANCC)

Pediatric Nursing Certifications:

- Certified Pediatric Nurse (CPN) through Pediatric Nursing Certification Board
- Child and Adolescent Psychiatric-Mental Health Clinical Nurse Specialist (PMHCNS-BC)

Specialized Certifications:

- Addiction nursing certification for those working with substance use disorders
- Forensic nursing certification for those in juvenile justice settings
- Trauma-informed care certifications from various organizations

Requirements and Benefits

Most certifications require:

- Current nursing license and specific education requirements
- Clinical experience in the specialty area
- Continuing education hours
- Passing a certification examination
- Periodic recertification through continuing education or re-examination

Benefits include:

- Higher salary potential (typically 5-15% increase)
- Professional recognition and credibility
- Career advancement opportunities
- Personal satisfaction and confidence
- Employer preference for certified nurses

Maintaining Certifications

Certification maintenance typically requires:

- Continuing education hours in the specialty area
- Evidence of ongoing clinical practice
- Professional development activities
- Some certifications require periodic re-examination

Continuing Education and Professional Development

The rapidly evolving field of pediatric mental health requires ongoing learning and skill development throughout one's career.

Formal Education Options

Graduate Degrees:

- Master's degrees in psychiatric nursing, counseling, or related fields
- Doctoral degrees (DNP or PhD) for advanced practice or research roles
- Post-master's certificates for additional specialization
- Dual degrees combining nursing with public health, business, or law

Certificate Programs:

- Trauma-informed care certificates
- Substance abuse treatment training
- Autism spectrum disorder specialization
- LGBTQ+ affirming care training

Professional Development Activities

Conferences and Workshops:

- American Psychiatric Nurses Association annual conferences
- International Association for Healthcare Communication and Marketing
- Specialized conferences on topics like trauma, autism, or adolescent development
- Local and regional professional meetings

Online Learning:

- Webinar series on current topics
- Self-paced online courses
- Virtual reality training simulations
- Massive open online courses (MOOCs) from universities

Professional Reading:

- Peer-reviewed journals in psychiatric nursing and pediatric mental health
- Professional magazines and newsletters
- Books on clinical topics, leadership, and personal development
- Research reports and white papers

Creating a Professional Development Plan

Effective professional development requires intentional planning:

Self-Assessment:

- Identify current strengths and areas for growth
- Consider career goals and interests
- Assess learning style preferences
- Evaluate available resources and constraints

Goal Setting:

- Establish specific, measurable learning objectives
- Set both short-term and long-term goals
- Align goals with career aspirations
- Consider personal and professional priorities

Resource Identification:

- Research available learning opportunities
- Consider costs and time commitments
- Identify potential mentors or colleagues
- Explore employer-supported development programs

Implementation and Evaluation:

- Create realistic timelines and schedules
- Track progress toward goals
- Adjust plans based on changing circumstances
- Evaluate outcomes and plan next steps

Think about James Wilson, a pediatric emergency department nurse who wanted to specialize in mental health. He started by taking online courses in crisis intervention, then volunteered to work extra shifts when psychiatric patients arrived. He pursued certification in psychiatric nursing while completing a master's degree part-time. Five years later, he became the clinical coordinator for psychiatric emergency services, a role that combined his emergency experience with his mental health specialization.

Mentorship and Career Guidance

Mentorship relationships can accelerate professional development and provide crucial support for navigating career challenges.

Types of Mentorship

Formal Mentorship Programs:

- Structured programs offered by employers or professional organizations
- Defined roles, expectations, and timelines
- Regular meetings and goal-setting activities
- Often include training for both mentors and mentees

Informal Mentorship:

- Naturally developing relationships with senior colleagues
- Flexible structure based on individual needs
- May focus on specific projects or challenges
- Can evolve over time as careers progress

Peer Mentorship:

- Mutual support relationships among colleagues at similar career stages
- Shared learning and problem-solving
- Professional networking and collaboration
- Can provide different perspectives and experiences

Reverse Mentorship:

- Younger professionals mentoring senior colleagues
- Often focuses on technology skills or cultural competency
- Mutually beneficial relationships
- Challenges traditional mentorship hierarchies

Finding Mentors

Within Your Organization:

- Senior nurses or advanced practice providers
- Supervisors and managers
- Colleagues in other departments or roles
- Medical staff or interdisciplinary team members

Professional Organizations:

- Networking events and conferences
- Mentorship matching programs
- Online professional communities
- Alumni networks from educational programs

External Networks:

- Social media professional groups
- Community leaders in mental health
- Researchers and academics
- Entrepreneurs and innovators

Being an Effective Mentee

Come Prepared:

- Have specific questions or topics to discuss
- Set clear goals and expectations
- Do homework between meetings
- Show initiative and follow-through

Show Appreciation:

- Respect mentors' time and expertise
- Express gratitude regularly
- Share updates on progress and achievements
- Offer assistance when appropriate

Take Ownership:

- Drive the relationship and schedule meetings
- Take responsibility for your own development
- Apply advice and feedback actively
- Learn from failures and setbacks

Becoming a Mentor

As professionals advance in their careers, becoming a mentor offers opportunities to give back while continuing to learn:

Benefits of Mentoring:

- Personal satisfaction from helping others succeed
- Learning new perspectives and approaches
- Building leadership and coaching skills
- Expanding professional networks
- Contributing to workforce development

Effective Mentoring Practices:

- Listen actively and ask thoughtful questions
- Share experiences and lessons learned
- Provide honest, constructive feedback
- Connect mentees with other resources and contacts
- Respect confidentiality and professional boundaries

Leadership Development in Pediatric Mental Health

The field desperately needs strong leaders who can address workforce challenges, improve care quality, and advocate for systemic changes.

Types of Leadership Roles

Clinical Leadership:

- Charge nurses and team leaders
- Clinical supervisors and coordinators
- Quality improvement champions
- Evidence-based practice leaders

Organizational Leadership:

- Department managers and directors
- Program coordinators and administrators

- Chief nursing officers and executives
- Board members and trustees

Professional Leadership:

- Professional organization officers
- Committee chairs and task force leaders
- Conference planners and speakers
- Journal editors and peer reviewers

Community Leadership:

- Community coalition members
- Public health advocates
- Policy influencers and lobbyists
- Media spokespersons and experts

Leadership Competencies

Personal Competencies:

- Self-awareness and emotional intelligence
- Resilience and stress management
- Ethical decision-making and integrity
- Continuous learning and adaptability

Interpersonal Competencies:

- Communication and active listening
- Conflict resolution and negotiation
- Team building and collaboration
- Mentoring and coaching others

Organizational Competencies:

- Strategic thinking and planning
- Change management and innovation
- Financial acumen and resource management

- Quality improvement and performance measurement

Systems Competencies:

- Understanding healthcare policy and regulation
- Building partnerships and coalitions
- Advocating for systemic change
- Influencing decision-makers and stakeholders

Developing Leadership Skills

Formal Leadership Development:

- Leadership courses and certificate programs
- Executive coaching and development programs
- MBA or other business education
- Leadership competency assessments

Experiential Learning:

- Volunteering for leadership roles and projects
- Cross-training in different departments or functions
- Serving on committees and task forces
- Leading quality improvement initiatives

Self-Directed Learning:

- Reading leadership and business books
- Following thought leaders and innovators
- Attending leadership conferences and seminars
- Practicing reflection and self-assessment

Consider Dr. Patricia Kim, who started as a staff nurse but always felt passionate about improving care systems. She volunteered to lead a medication safety initiative, which led to opportunities to chair the quality committee and eventually become director of nursing. Through each role, she focused on developing her leadership skills while maintaining her commitment to direct patient care.

Research and Evidence-Based Practice

Contributing to the knowledge base in pediatric mental health through research and evidence-based practice initiatives can be deeply rewarding while advancing the field.

Types of Research Opportunities

Clinical Research:

- Intervention studies testing new treatments or approaches
- Outcome studies measuring effectiveness of existing programs
- Comparative effectiveness research examining different treatment options
- Implementation science studying how to best implement evidence-based practices

Health Services Research:

- Access and quality studies examining healthcare delivery
- Health economics research on costs and cost-effectiveness
- Health policy research on regulations and legislation
- Workforce studies examining provider shortage and satisfaction

Quality Improvement Research:

- Process improvement studies within specific organizations
- Patient safety research identifying and addressing risks
- Performance measurement studies developing and testing quality indicators
- Implementation research supporting practice changes

Getting Involved in Research

Starting Small:

- Participate in quality improvement projects
- Collect and analyze data for program evaluation
- Conduct literature reviews on topics of interest
- Present findings at local or regional meetings

Building Skills:

- Take research methods courses
- Learn statistical analysis software
- Attend research conferences and workshops
- Find research mentors and collaborators

Formal Opportunities:

- Join research teams as data collectors or coordinators
- Apply for research fellowships or training grants
- Pursue doctoral education with research focus
- Collaborate with academic institutions on projects

Implementing Evidence-Based Practice

Staying Current:

- Regularly review professional literature
- Participate in journal clubs and case discussions
- Attend conferences focusing on evidence-based practice
- Use clinical practice guidelines and recommendations

Leading Change:

- Champion implementation of new evidence-based interventions
- Develop protocols and procedures based on current evidence
- Mentor colleagues in evidence-based practice approaches
- Measure and share outcomes from practice changes

Think about Dr. Michael Torres, a nurse practitioner who noticed that many of his adolescent patients weren't responding well to traditional therapy approaches. He began researching dialectical behavior therapy for adolescents and eventually led implementation of a DBT program at his clinic. The success of this program led to opportunities to present at conferences, publish papers, and consult with other organizations wanting to implement similar programs.

Self-Care and Resilience

Working in pediatric mental health can be emotionally demanding, making self-care and resilience-building essential for long-term career success and personal wellbeing.

Understanding Secondary Trauma and Burnout

Secondary Traumatic Stress: Emotional duress experienced by persons as a result of exposure to a trauma survivor, often called "compassion fatigue."

Symptoms may include:

- Intrusive thoughts about clients' traumatic experiences
- Avoidance of certain types of clients or cases
- Negative changes in mood and thinking
- Sleep disturbances and physical symptoms
- Hypervigilance and anxiety

Professional Burnout: A psychological syndrome emerging as a prolonged response to chronic interpersonal stressors on the job.

Components include:

- Emotional exhaustion and depletion
- Depersonalization and cynicism toward clients
- Reduced sense of personal accomplishment
- Physical symptoms and health problems

Risk and Protective Factors

Individual Risk Factors:

- Personal trauma history
- Perfectionism and high expectations
- Poor work-life balance
- Limited coping skills
- Social isolation

Organizational Risk Factors:

- High caseloads and time pressures
- Lack of supervision and support
- Limited resources and funding
- Workplace conflict and tension
- Unclear roles and expectations

Protective Factors:

- Strong personal support systems
- Effective coping and stress management skills
- Meaningful work and sense of purpose
- Professional development opportunities
- Organizational support and recognition

Self-Care Strategies

Physical Self-Care:

- Regular exercise and movement
- Adequate sleep and nutrition
- Medical and dental care
- Relaxation and stress reduction techniques
- Limiting caffeine and alcohol consumption

Emotional Self-Care:

- Personal therapy or counseling
- Journaling and reflection
- Creative expression and hobbies
- Mindfulness and meditation practices
- Maintaining friendships and social connections

Professional Self-Care:

- Setting appropriate boundaries with clients
- Seeking supervision and consultation
- Continuing education and skill development
- Professional networking and peer support
- Taking vacation time and breaks

Spiritual Self-Care:

- Connecting with personal values and meaning
- Participating in religious or spiritual practices
- Spending time in nature
- Practicing gratitude and appreciation
- Contributing to causes larger than oneself

Building Resilience

Individual Resilience:

- Developing optimism and hope
- Building problem-solving skills
- Cultivating flexibility and adaptability
- Practicing self-compassion
- Learning from setbacks and failures

Professional Resilience:

- Finding meaning and purpose in work
- Building competence and confidence
- Developing professional identity
- Creating supportive colleague relationships

- Maintaining perspective on successes and challenges

Organizational Resilience:

- Creating cultures of support and collaboration
- Providing resources for staff wellbeing
- Recognizing and addressing workplace stress
- Supporting professional development
- Celebrating achievements and milestones

Remember Sarah from our opening story? She realized that her struggle wasn't a sign of weakness but a natural response to challenging work. She started seeing her own therapist, joined a peer support group for psychiatric nurses, and worked with her supervisor to adjust her caseload. She also began leading a mindfulness group for staff, which helped both her colleagues and her own wellbeing. Two years later, she was promoted to clinical supervisor and became a mentor for new psychiatric nurses.

Advocacy and Policy Engagement

Pediatric mental health professionals have unique insights into system challenges and opportunities, making their voices essential in policy and advocacy efforts.

Types of Advocacy

Individual Advocacy:

- Advocating for specific patients and families
- Helping families navigate healthcare and educational systems
- Connecting families with resources and supports
- Supporting families in legal or administrative proceedings

Professional Advocacy:

- Promoting nursing profession recognition and autonomy

- Supporting scope of practice expansions
- Advocating for fair reimbursement and working conditions
- Promoting nursing education and workforce development

System Advocacy:

- Supporting mental health parity legislation
- Advocating for increased mental health funding
- Promoting policy changes to improve care access and quality
- Supporting research funding and priorities

Social Justice Advocacy:

- Addressing healthcare disparities and inequities
- Supporting vulnerable and marginalized populations
- Promoting social determinants of health approaches
- Advocating for human rights and dignity

Getting Involved in Policy

Local Level:

- Participating in community coalitions and task forces
- Attending city council or school board meetings
- Writing letters to local newspapers
- Volunteering for local candidates or causes

State Level:

- Joining professional organization advocacy committees
- Participating in lobby days and legislative visits
- Providing testimony at legislative hearings
- Building relationships with state legislators and staff

National Level:

- Contacting federal representatives about national issues
- Participating in national professional organization advocacy

- Submitting comments on federal regulations
- Engaging in social media advocacy campaigns

Effective Advocacy Strategies

Know Your Issues:

- Stay informed about current policy debates and proposals
- Understand how policies affect children, families, and providers
- Learn about the legislative and regulatory processes
- Identify key decision-makers and influencers

Tell Your Story:

- Share personal and professional experiences
- Use specific examples and concrete outcomes
- Explain complex issues in understandable terms
- Connect policy changes to real-world impacts

Build Relationships:

- Develop ongoing relationships with policymakers and staff
- Participate in professional organizations and coalitions
- Collaborate with other healthcare professionals and advocates
- Maintain regular communication, not just during crises

Be Strategic:

- Choose issues that align with your expertise and passion
- Time advocacy efforts for maximum impact
- Use data and evidence to support your positions
- Consider multiple approaches and tactics

Think about Dr. Linda Washington, who became frustrated with insurance denials for evidence-based treatments. She started by advocating for individual patients, then joined her professional organization's advocacy committee. Eventually, she testified before the state legislature about mental health parity issues and helped draft regulations requiring insurance coverage for specific pediatric mental health services.

Building Professional Networks

Strong professional networks provide support, opportunities, and resources throughout your career.

Types of Professional Networks

Workplace Networks:

- Colleagues in your organization
- Interdisciplinary team members
- Leaders and supervisors
- Mentors and mentees

Professional Organization Networks:

- Professional association members
- Committee and task force participants
- Conference attendees and speakers
- Online community members

Educational Networks:

- Former classmates and faculty
- Continuing education participants
- Research collaborators
- Academic partners

Community Networks:

- Local healthcare professionals
- Community organization leaders
- Volunteer and advocacy partners

- Social and recreational connections

Building and Maintaining Networks

Be Genuine:

- Focus on building real relationships, not just collecting contacts
- Show authentic interest in others' work and experiences
- Offer help and support before asking for assistance
- Follow through on commitments and promises

Stay Connected:

- Maintain regular contact with network members
- Share updates on your professional activities
- Congratulate others on achievements and milestones
- Offer condolences and support during difficult times

Give Back:

- Mentor newer professionals
- Share knowledge and resources
- Make introductions and connections for others
- Volunteer for professional organizations and causes

Use Technology:

- Maintain professional social media profiles
- Participate in online professional communities
- Use networking apps and platforms
- Share relevant content and resources

Entrepreneurship and Innovation

The pediatric mental health field needs innovative solutions to address workforce shortages, improve care quality, and expand access to services.

Types of Entrepreneurial Opportunities

Clinical Innovation:

- Developing new treatment approaches or protocols
- Creating specialized programs for specific populations
- Implementing technology-enhanced interventions
- Designing care delivery models

Educational Innovation:

- Developing training programs and curricula
- Creating educational resources and tools
- Implementing simulation and technology-enhanced learning
- Providing consultation and technical assistance

Technology Innovation:

- Developing mental health apps and platforms
- Creating assessment and monitoring tools
- Implementing artificial intelligence and machine learning solutions
- Designing virtual reality and gaming interventions

Business Model Innovation:

- Creating new practice models and structures
- Developing sustainable financing approaches
- Implementing value-based payment models
- Creating partnerships and collaborations

Entrepreneurial Skills and Competencies

Innovation and Creativity:

- Identifying unmet needs and opportunities
- Generating novel solutions to complex problems
- Thinking outside traditional approaches

- Learning from failure and iteration

Business Acumen:

- Understanding financial management and planning
- Developing business plans and strategies
- Marketing and promotion skills
- Legal and regulatory knowledge

Leadership and Management:

- Building and leading teams
- Managing projects and timelines
- Communicating vision and strategy
- Adapting to change and uncertainty

Risk Management:

- Assessing and managing financial risks
- Understanding legal and professional liability
- Planning for contingencies and setbacks
- Balancing innovation with safety

Consider Dr. Amanda Foster, who noticed that many rural families couldn't access specialized autism services for their children. She developed a telehealth program that connected families with autism specialists and trained local providers to deliver interventions. Her program expanded to serve multiple states and became a model for other rural mental health initiatives.

Preparing for the Future

The pediatric mental health field will continue evolving rapidly, requiring professionals to stay adaptable and forward-thinking.

Emerging Trends and Opportunities

Technology Integration:

- Artificial intelligence and machine learning applications
- Virtual and augmented reality interventions
- Wearable devices and remote monitoring
- Digital therapeutics and precision medicine

Care Model Evolution:

- Integrated and collaborative care approaches
- Prevention and early intervention focus
- Community-based and school-based services
- Peer support and family engagement models

Workforce Development:

- New roles and specializations
- Team-based care approaches
- Task-shifting and delegation strategies
- International recruitment and exchange programs

Policy and Regulation Changes:

- Mental health parity enforcement
- Telehealth regulation and reimbursement
- Scope of practice expansions
- Quality measurement and value-based payment

Preparing for Change

Stay Informed:

- Follow industry trends and developments
- Participate in professional organizations and conferences
- Read professional literature and research
- Engage with thought leaders and innovators

Develop Adaptability:

- Cultivate growth mindset and learning orientation

- Build resilience and change management skills
- Practice flexibility in approaches and solutions
- Embrace experimentation and iteration

Build Diverse Skills:

- Develop technology literacy and comfort
- Learn business and entrepreneurship skills
- Build cultural competency and global awareness
- Strengthen leadership and communication abilities

Create Support Systems:

- Build strong professional networks
- Develop mentoring relationships
- Participate in peer support groups
- Maintain personal wellness and resilience

Your Leadership Journey

Every pediatric mental health professional has the potential to be a leader, whether through direct patient care excellence, system improvements, research contributions, or policy advocacy.

Leadership isn't just about formal titles or positions—it's about making a positive difference in the lives of children and families while contributing to the growth and improvement of the field. Some professionals will lead through clinical innovation, developing new approaches to treatment and care. Others will lead through education, preparing the next generation of providers. Still others will lead through research, generating new knowledge that improves outcomes.

The field needs all types of leaders: the bedside nurse who advocates fiercely for their patients, the nurse practitioner who implements evidence-based practices, the administrator who creates supportive work environments, the educator who inspires students, the researcher who discovers new interventions, and the policy advocate who fights for systemic change.

Your leadership journey will be unique to your interests, skills, and circumstances. But whatever path you choose, remember that leadership in pediatric mental health is ultimately about hope—hope for healing, hope for better systems, hope for stronger communities, and hope for a future where every child has access to the mental health support they need to thrive.

Sarah's story, which began this chapter with burnout and despair, evolved into one of growth and leadership. She learned to care for herself while caring for others, developed skills in supervision and mentoring, and eventually became a voice for system improvements. Her journey from struggling new practitioner to confident leader illustrates that challenges can become catalysts for growth when approached with intentionality and support.

The pediatric mental health field needs professionals who are committed to their own development while remaining focused on the ultimate goal: helping children and families heal and thrive. With the right combination of clinical skills, leadership development, self-care, and professional support, you can build a sustainable, meaningful career that makes a lasting difference in the lives of those you serve.

Essential Tools for Success

Professional Development Planning Template

Self-Assessment:

- Current skills and competencies
- Areas for growth and development
- Career interests and values
- Learning style preferences

Goal Setting:

- Short-term objectives (6-12 months)
- Medium-term goals (2-3 years)
- Long-term vision (5-10 years)
- Personal and professional priorities

Action Planning:

- Specific learning activities and experiences
- Timeline and milestones
- Resources and support needed
- Success measures and evaluation methods

Self-Care Assessment and Planning

Current Status:

- Physical health and wellness
- Emotional and mental wellbeing
- Professional satisfaction and engagement
- Personal relationships and social support

Risk Factors:

- Work-related stressors and challenges
- Personal vulnerabilities and triggers
- Environmental and organizational factors
- Life circumstances and changes

Self-Care Strategies:

- Daily self-care practices
- Weekly restoration activities
- Monthly professional development
- Annual renewal and planning

Leadership Development Resources

Books and Reading:

- Leadership and management texts
- Biographies of inspiring leaders
- Professional development resources
- Industry and healthcare literature

Training and Education:

- Leadership courses and workshops
- Professional conferences and seminars
- Online learning platforms
- Academic degree programs

Experiential Learning:

- Volunteer leadership opportunities
- Committee and task force participation
- Mentoring and coaching relationships
- Cross-functional projects and assignments

The pediatric mental health field offers tremendous opportunities for professionals who approach their careers with intention, dedication, and a commitment to lifelong learning. By focusing on professional development, building supportive relationships, maintaining personal wellness, and contributing to the advancement of the field, you can create a career that is both personally fulfilling and professionally impactful.

The children and families we serve deserve our very best—skilled, compassionate, resilient professionals who are committed to their own growth and the improvement of the systems in which we work. Your journey in pediatric mental health has the potential to transform not only your own life but the lives of countless children and families who need our support, expertise, and advocacy.

References

- Achenbach, T. M., & Rescorla, L. A. (2001). *Manual for the ASEBA School-Age Forms & Profiles*. University of Vermont, Research Center for Children, Youth, & Families.

- Ainsworth, M. D. S., Blehar, M. C., Waters, E., & Wall, S. (1978). *Patterns of attachment: A psychological study of the strange situation*. Lawrence Erlbaum Associates.

- American Academy of Child and Adolescent Psychiatry. (2008). Practice parameter for telepsychiatry with children and adolescents. *Journal of the American Academy of Child & Adolescent Psychiatry*, 47(12), 1468–1483. https://doi.org/10.1097/CHI.0b013e31818b4e13

- American Association of Colleges of Nursing. (2021). *The Essentials: Core Competencies for Professional Nursing Education*. AACN.

- American Organization for Nursing Leadership. (2020). *Nurse Manager Competencies*. AONL.

- American Psychiatric Association. (2022). *Diagnostic and statistical manual of mental disorders* (5th ed., text rev.). American Psychiatric Publishing.

- APNA; ISPN; & American Nurses Association. (2022). *Psychiatric–Mental Health Nursing: Scope and Standards of Practice* (latest ed.). American Nurses Association.

- Bandura, A. (1977). *Social learning theory*. Prentice Hall.

- Beck, A. J., Page, C., Buche, J., Rittman, D., & Gaiser, M. (2019). *Estimating the distribution of the U.S. psychiatric subspecialist workforce*. University of Michigan Behavioral Health Workforce Research Center.

- Beck, A. T. (1976). *Cognitive therapy and the emotional disorders*. International Universities Press.

- Birmaher, B., Brent, D. A., Chiappetta, L., Bridge, J., Monga, S., & Baugher, M. (1999). Psychometric properties of the Screen for Child Anxiety Related Emotional Disorders (SCARED): A replication study. *Journal of the American Academy of Child & Adolescent Psychiatry*, 38(10), 1230–1236. https://doi.org/10.1097/00004583-199910000-00011

- Bowlby, J. (1969). *Attachment and loss: Vol. 1. Attachment.* Basic Books.

- Bronfenbrenner, U. (1979). *The ecology of human development*. Harvard University Press.

- Cohen, J. A., Mannarino, A. P., Kliethermes, M., & Murray, L. A. (2012). Trauma-focused CBT for youth with complex trauma. *Child Abuse & Neglect*, 36(6), 528–541. https://doi.org/10.1016/j.chiabu.2012.03.007

- Cohen, J. A., Mannarino, A. P., & Deblinger, E. (2017). *Treating trauma and traumatic grief in children and adolescents* (2nd ed.). Guilford Press.

- Crenshaw, D. A., & Stewart, A. L. (Eds.). (2015). *Play therapy: A comprehensive guide to theory and practice*. Guilford Press.

- De Hert, M., Dobbelaere, M., Sheridan, E. M., Cohen, D., & Correll, C. U. (2011). Metabolic and endocrine adverse effects of second-generation antipsychotics in children and adolescents: A systematic review of randomized, placebo-controlled trials and guidelines for clinical practice. *European Psychiatry*, 26(3), 144–158. https://doi.org/10.1016/j.eurpsy.2010.09.011

- Erikson, E. H. (1968). *Identity: Youth and crisis*. W. W. Norton & Company.

- Felitti, V. J., Anda, R. F., Nordenberg, D., Williamson, D. F., Spitz, A. M., Edwards, V., Koss, M. P., & Marks, J. S. (1998). Relationship of childhood abuse and household dysfunction to many of the leading causes of death in adults: The Adverse Childhood Experiences (ACE) Study. *American Journal of Preventive Medicine*, 14(4), 245–258. https://doi.org/10.1016/S0749-3797(98)00017-8

- Figley, C. R. (2002). Compassion fatigue: Psychotherapists' chronic lack of self-care. *Journal of Clinical Psychology*, 58(11), 1433–1441. https://doi.org/10.1002/jclp.10090

- Goodman, R. (1997). The Strengths and Difficulties Questionnaire: A research note. *Journal of Child Psychology and Psychiatry*, 38(5), 581–586. https://doi.org/10.1111/j.1469-7610.1997.tb01545.x

- Horowitz, L. M., Bridge, J. A., Teach, S. J., Ballard, E., Klima, J., Rosenstein, D. L., Wharff, E. A., Ginnis, K., Cannon, E., Joshi, P., Pao, M., & Carl, R. (2012). Ask Suicide-Screening Questions (ASQ): A brief instrument for the pediatric emergency department. *Archives of Pediatrics & Adolescent Medicine*, 166(12), 1170–1176. https://doi.org/10.1001/archpediatrics.2012.1276

- Institute of Medicine. (2011). *The future of nursing: Leading change, advancing health*. The National Academies Press.

- Jobes, D. A. (2016). *Managing suicidal risk: A collaborative approach* (2nd ed.). Guilford Press.

- Kaufman, J., Birmaher, B., Brent, D., Rao, U., Flynn, C., Moreci, P., Williamson, D., & Ryan, N. (1997). Schedule for Affective Disorders and Schizophrenia for School-Age Children—Present and Lifetime Version (K-SADS-PL): Initial reliability and validity data. *Journal of the American*

Academy of Child & Adolescent Psychiatry, 36(7), 980–988.
https://doi.org/10.1097/00004583-199707000-00021

- Kendall, P. C. (Ed.). (2012). *Child and adolescent therapy: Cognitive-behavioral procedures* (4th ed.). Guilford Press.

- Knight, J. R., Sherritt, L., Shrier, L. A., Harris, S. K., & Chang, G. (2002). Validity of the CRAFFT substance abuse screening test among adolescent clinic patients. *Archives of Pediatrics & Adolescent Medicine*, 156(6), 607–614. https://doi.org/10.1001/archpedi.156.6.607

- Kroenke, K., Spitzer, R. L., & Williams, J. B. (2001). The PHQ-9: Validity of a brief depression severity measure. *Journal of General Internal Medicine*, 16(9), 606–613. https://doi.org/10.1046/j.1525-1497.2001.016009606.x

- Linehan, M. M. (1993). *Cognitive-behavioral treatment of borderline personality disorder*. Guilford Press.

- Linehan, M. M., Rathus, J. H., & Miller, A. L. (2015). *DBT skills manual for adolescents*. Guilford Press.

- Lord, C., Rutter, M., DiLavore, P. C., Risi, S., Gotham, K., & Bishop, S. L. (2012). *Autism Diagnostic Observation Schedule, Second Edition (ADOS-2)*. Western Psychological Services.

- March, J. S., Parker, J. D., Sullivan, K., Stallings, P., & Conners, C. K. (1997). The Multidimensional Anxiety Scale for Children (MASC): Factor structure, reliability, and validity. *Journal of the American Academy of Child & Adolescent Psychiatry*, 36(4), 554–565. https://doi.org/10.1097/00004583-199704000-00019

- McCabe, R., & Priebe, S. (2004). The therapeutic relationship in the treatment of severe mental illness: A review of methods and findings. *International Journal of*

Social Psychiatry, 50(2), 115–128.
https://doi.org/10.1177/0020764004040959

- Merikangas, K. R., He, J. P., Burstein, M., Swanson, S. A., Avenevoli, S., Cui, L., Benjet, C., Georgiades, K., & Swendsen, J. (2010). Lifetime prevalence of mental disorders in U.S. adolescents: Results from the National Comorbidity Survey Replication–Adolescent Supplement (NCS-A). *Journal of the American Academy of Child & Adolescent Psychiatry*, 49(10), 980–989. https://doi.org/10.1016/j.jaac.2010.05.017

- National Academies of Sciences, Engineering, and Medicine. (2019). *Taking action against clinician burnout: A systems approach to professional well-being.* National Academies Press. https://doi.org/10.17226/25521

- Olfson, M., King, M., & Schoenbaum, M. (2015). Treatment of young people with antipsychotic medications in the United States. *JAMA Psychiatry*, 72(9), 867–874. https://doi.org/10.1001/jamapsychiatry.2015.0500

- Posner, K., Brown, G. K., Stanley, B., Brent, D. A., Yershova, K. V., Oquendo, M. A., Currier, G. W., Melvin, G., Greenhill, L., Shen, S., & Mann, J. J. (2011). The Columbia–Suicide Severity Rating Scale: Initial validity and internal consistency findings from three multisite studies with adolescents and adults. *American Journal of Psychiatry*, 168(12), 1266–1277. https://doi.org/10.1176/appi.ajp.2011.10111704

- Price, M., Spinazzola, J., Musicaro, R., Turner, J., Suvak, M., Emerson, D., & van der Kolk, B. (2017). Effectiveness of an extended yoga treatment for women with chronic posttraumatic stress disorder. *Journal of Alternative and Complementary Medicine*, 23(4), 300–309. https://doi.org/10.1089/acm.2016.0103

- Rathus, J. H., & Miller, A. L. (2014). *DBT skills manual for adolescents with emotion dysregulation.* Guilford Press.

- Reynolds, C. R., & Kamphaus, R. W. (2015). *Behavior Assessment System for Children* (3rd ed.). Pearson.

- Robins, D. L., Casagrande, K., Barton, M., Chen, C.-M. A., Dumont-Mathieu, T., & Fein, D. (2014). Validation of the Modified Checklist for Autism in Toddlers, Revised With Follow-Up (M-CHAT-R/F). *Pediatrics*, 133(1), 37–45. https://doi.org/10.1542/peds.2013-1813 *(Corrects earlier "self-published 2009" entry.)*

- SAMHSA. (2014). *Trauma-Informed Care in Behavioral Health Services* (Treatment Improvement Protocol [TIP] Series 57; HHS Publication No. SMA 13-4801). Substance Abuse and Mental Health Services Administration. *(Common PDF file code "SMA14-4816.")*

- Spitzer, R. L., Kroenke, K., Williams, J. B., & Löwe, B. (2006). A brief measure for assessing generalized anxiety disorder: The GAD-7. *Archives of Internal Medicine*, 166(10), 1092–1097. https://doi.org/10.1001/archinte.166.10.1092

- Squires, J., & Bricker, D. (2009). *Ages & Stages Questionnaires* (3rd ed.). Paul H. Brookes Publishing.

- Stanley, B., & Brown, G. K. (2012). Safety planning intervention: A brief intervention to mitigate suicide risk. *Cognitive and Behavioral Practice*, 19(2), 256–264. https://doi.org/10.1016/j.cbpra.2011.01.001

- Stanley, B., Brown, G. K., Brenner, L. A., Galfalvy, H. C., Currier, G. W., Knox, K. L., Chaudhury, S. R., Busch, A. B., & Green, K. L. (2018). Comparison of the safety planning intervention with follow-up vs usual care of suicidal patients treated in the emergency department. *JAMA Psychiatry*,

75(9), 894–900.
https://doi.org/10.1001/jamapsychiatry.2018.1776

- Twenge, J. M., & Campbell, W. K. (2018). Associations between screen time and lower psychological well-being among children and adolescents: Evidence from a population-based study. *Preventive Medicine Reports*, 12, 271–283. https://doi.org/10.1016/j.pmedr.2018.10.003 *(Corrects journal title/series.)*

- van der Kolk, B. A., Stone, L., West, J., Rhodes, A., Emerson, D., Suvak, M., & Spinazzola, J. (2014). Yoga as an adjunctive treatment for posttraumatic stress disorder: A randomized controlled trial. *Journal of Clinical Psychiatry*, 75(6), e559–e565. https://doi.org/10.4088/JCP.13m08561 *(Corrects pagination to e-pages.)*

- Walkup, J. T., Albano, A. M., Piacentini, J., Birmaher, B., Compton, S. N., Sherrill, J. T., Ginsburg, G., Rynn, M. A., McCracken, J., Waslick, B. D., Iyengar, S., March, J. S., & Kendall, P. C. (2008). Cognitive behavioral therapy, sertraline, or a combination in childhood anxiety. *New England Journal of Medicine*, 359(26), 2753–2766. https://doi.org/10.1056/NEJMoa0804633

- Weisz, J. R., Kazdin, A. E., & Kendall, P. C. (Eds.). (2017). *Evidence-based psychotherapies for children and adolescents* (3rd ed.). Guilford Press.

- Wharff, E. A., Ginnis, K. M., Ross, A. M., & Blood, E. A. (2019). Family-based crisis intervention with suicidal adolescents: A randomized clinical trial. *Pediatric Emergency Care*, 35(3), 170–175. https://doi.org/10.1097/PEC.0000000000001068

- World Health Organization. (2022). *World mental health report: Transforming mental health for all*. WHO.

- Wolraich, M. L., Lambert, W., Doffing, M. A., Bickman, L., Simmons, T., & Worley, K. (2003). Psychometric properties of the Vanderbilt ADHD diagnostic parent rating scale in a referred population. *Journal of Pediatric Psychology*, 28(8), 559–568. https://doi.org/10.1093/jpepsy/jsg046

- Youngstrom, E. A., & Prinstein, M. J. (Eds.). (2020). *Assessment of disorders in childhood and adolescence* (5th ed.). Guilford Press.

- Zero to Three. (2016). *DC:0–5™ Diagnostic classification of mental health and developmental disorders of infancy and early childhood*. Zero to Three.

- Zwaanswijk, M., Verhaak, P. F., Bensing, J. M., van der Ende, J., & Verhulst, F. C. (2003). Help seeking for emotional and behavioural problems in children and adolescents. *European Child & Adolescent Psychiatry*, 12(4), 153–161. https://doi.org/10.1007/s00787-003-0322-6

www.ingramcontent.com/pod-product-compliance
Lightning Source LLC
Chambersburg PA
CBHW061002280326
41935CB00009B/799